Using God's Medicine for the Abundant Life

An Evidence-Based Approach to Essential Oils

By Eric L. Zielinski, DC, MPH(c)

|© 2016 | Biblical Health Publishing |

Printed in the Unite States of America
First Printing, 2015

ISBN - 13: 978-0-9971655-1-7

Biblical Health Publishing
2774 N. Cobb Pkwy
Suite 109-389
Kennesaw, GA 30152

www.BiblicalHealthPublishing.com

Ordering Information:

Quantity sales. Special discounts are available on quantity purchases by corporations, churches, and others. For details contact publisher at Orders@BiblicalHealthPublishing

Printed in the United States of America

Contents

Introduction

"And the leaves of the trees are for the healing of the nations."
~ Rev 22:2

I truly believe that *essential oils are God's Medicine.* It's not that we need science to validate what God has set in motion before time began, but it's nice to have some research to support what folk medicine has practiced with great success for over 3,500 years. Scientists are just now tapping into how powerful essential oils are to cure all types of diseases and to help people live the Abundant Life.

This book was designed to help you sift through all this data and to provide you with practical uses that can easily be implemented today. Essentially, this book is an anthology, and my suggestion is that you don't read it cover to cover. Take in each chapter as your interest and need dictates; embrace the journey.

George Bernard Shaw once said, *"Progress is impossible without change, and those who cannot change their minds cannot change anything."* I have not always been an essential oil enthusiast. In fact, I was pretty clueless to their profound health benefits until I met my wife several years ago. After dabbling on my own for a while, I wasn't too impressed until I started digging into the scientific literature. And then I got convicted. It dawned on me that I was literally poisoning myself with conventional personal use and body care products, and I started to look for "alternatives." Ironically, I discovered that these so-called alternatives are the real-deal and that they should be our first choice from the get-go.

If you're anything like me, some of the information presented here will challenge your current health care paradigm, and that's a good thing. Please stop by my website (www.DrEricZ.com) and leave a comment or two so we can hash it out together!

~Dr. Z

How to Safely Use Essential Oils

Pure therapeutic grade essential oils can be used safely by your family for a variety of wellness applications. However, there are several safety guidelines that you should follow when using essential oils and essential oil products.

- Remember, a little goes a long way.
- Be sure to use only pure, therapeutic-grade essential oils and follow all label warnings and instructions.
- For topical use, always dilute essential oils with a carrier oil such as fractionated coconut oil, jojoba, or almond oil.
- Essential oils should not be used in the eyes, inside the ear canal, or in open wounds. In the event of accidental contact with the eye, dilute with a carrier oil.
- Do NOT consume an essential oil internally unless labeled with a Supplement Facts box that includes specific dietary supplement, use instructions, and warnings.
- Never take more than a few drops in a gel cap, and never take more that 1 or 2 drops in water at one time.
- Discontinue the use of an essential oil if you experience severe skin, stomach, esophageal & respiratory irritation, or discomfort.
- When using on children, heavily dilute essential oils. Apply a very small amount of the oil to test skin or other sensitivity. Do not use oil on a child's hand as they may transfer to their eyes or mouth.
- Consult your physician before using essential oils if you are pregnant or under a doctor's care, or have other safety questions regarding essential oils.

Lastly, it is important to remember that therapeutic-grade essential oils are highly-concentrated plant extracts, and should be used with reasonable care. Consulting with someone who has experience with essential oils will make your first experience with them more enjoyable and rewarding. As you learn how to use essential oils through personal experience, share your knowledge with others in a safe and responsible way and encourage others to do the same.

Daily Essential Oils User Guide

We have been using essential oils for years. I'm actually a late-bloomer compared to my wife, Sabrina, who has been using them since she was in her teens! We've tried all the brands and have completely rearranged our medicine cabinets over the years.

For those of you who want to start using essential oils but don't know where to start, here's a **Daily Essential Oils User Guide** that you and your family can start using today!

Morning Immune Booster

Arguably the most potent medicinal EO out there, recent research studies suggest that frankincense not only kills cancer cells, but it also promotes health and vitality in neighboring non-cancerous cells! To help prevent getting sick and boost your immune system, simply:

- Add 1 drop of frankincense to a tsp of honey, maple syrup, or coonut oil. Take first thing in the morning. You can also add 1 drop to 4 oz of water and drink.

Oil Pulling

Oil pulling works by detoxifying your oral cavity in a similar way that soap cleans dirty dishes. Because most toxins are fat-soluble, it literally sucks the dirt (toxins) out of your mouth and creates an antiseptic oral environment that contributes to the proper flow of dental liquid that is needed to prevent cavities and disease. The ancient Ayurvedic system for health in India has used oil pulling for years to treat just under 30 systemic diseases, ranging from headaches and tooth decay to diabetes and asthma.

To help detox and keep your smile bright and shining, mix essential oils with unrefined, organic coconut oil. Here are some tips:

- Like most other detoxification procedures, the best time to oil pull is first thing in the morning, right after you get out of bed.
- All you need to do is swish between 1 – 2 tablespoons of the coconut or sesame oil and essential oil in your mouth for 20 minutes. Easy peasy!
- Don't worry, you won't even notice 20 minutes have gone by if you do this during your normal morning routine (i.e. while you shower, put your clothes on, and prep for the day).
- Immediately afterward, rinse your mouth out with warm water.
- Use salt water for added antimicrobial properties.
- Don't be shocked if the oil/saliva mixture you spit out is milky white or yellow.
- Finally, brush your teeth as normal.

Note: This should be a relatively relaxing process, so don't think that you need to swish your mouth with oil for the entire time – you'll be bound to wear out your jaw muscles! Simply move the oil in your mouth and through your teeth without swallowing any of it.

Oil Pulling & EO Applications: I recommend oil pulling no more than 3-4x per week.

- Add **1 drop each of clove** & **orange**, or **lemon** & **peppermint** with 1 tablespoon of coconut oil. If you're battling an infection, you may want to would change it up and use 2 drops of **an immunity blend** as a holistic remedy.

Oral Care

In addition to oil pulling, try using EO instead of (or in addition to toothpaste). One drop of **clove**, **peppermint,** or **orange** on your toothbrush will supercharge your fluoride-free toothpaste, or if you want to make your own remineralizing toothpaste, just combine Himalayan pink sea salt, baking soda, unrefined coconut oil and essential oils. Some of our favorite combinations are:

- **Sweet orange, grapefruit and lemon**
- **Peppermint, eucalyptus and melaleuca**
- **Clove, sweet orange and peppermint**

Body Care

Put 5 drops each of **eucalyptus**, **peppermint**, **melaleuca**, and **lavender** in 1 cup unrefined coconut oil. This is a fantastic natural anti-fungal, antibacterial mixture that works great as a lotion for the entire body and can substitute for deodorant.

Aromatherapy

Throw away the glade plug-ins and wall flowers! They emit toxic chemicals that have been linked to neurotoxicity and cancer, which is why every house should have multiple diffusers running throughout the day. Not only will they help make your house smell and feel refreshing, but they also emit aromatic essential oil "volatiles" that have significant medicinal properties. Research studies have linked inhaling diffused **lavender** EO to:

- Decreased oxidative stress
- Reduced postnatal depression and anxiety
- Improved mood for people suffering with PTSD
- Enhanced sleep and decreased moodiness
- Increased overall health status
- Prevented allergic reactions

Applying diluted **lavender** EO directly on cuts and burns has also been shown to speed would healing. On a personal note, I have extremely sensitive skin, and I have a tendency to nick myself pretty good when I shave my face. Whenever this happens, I put a drop of diluted **lavender** on my cut and the bleeding usually stops immediately!

- For burns or eczema, mix **lavender** with coconut oil in a 1:5 ratio to speed up the healing process.
- For sunburn or dry skin, add 5 drops of **lavender** in 1 ounce of aloe vera or coconut oil.

Remember: Quality NOT Quantity is Key!

One thing to remember is that not all essential oils are created equal. In fact, many on the market are veritably worthless to your health because they are over processed, include synthetic ingredients and are not organic. When buying essential oils, make sure they are a pure, therapeutic grade.

Top 10 Essential Oils for Healing

Essential oils are extracted directly from the bark, flower fruit, leaves, nut, resin or root of a plant or tree, and just one drop can provide the amazing health benefits that each oil provides. Used medicinally for thousands of years, the potency behind these oils is their ability to support your natural healing systems.

Essential oils are comprised of a complex network of molecules that each carry different effects to the body. Scientists can analyze the structure of an essential oil using gas chromatography/mass spectronomy (GC/MS) methods that reveal each molecular component.

Their power to heal and cure disease is so effective that, under the supervision of a natural health expert and herbalist, you could avoid the need to use a plethora of drugs or have various types of surgeries.

History of Essential Oils

Truth be told, essential oils as we know them today are very new on the scene of plant-based therapies. To be fair, ancient civilizations did employ crude distillations techniques, but the essential oils that were extracted centuries ago were a far cry from the potent, filtered, and pure compounds that we see on the market currently. The same is true with extracts, salves and poultices that were made from healing plants. They all contained essential oils and were, thus, very effective at preventing and managing disease. However, they definitely lacked the medicinal strength of oils that we use today.

Be that as it may, a vital component of ancient culture spanning at least 3,000 years, it appears that essential oils were enjoyed by those in ancient **Cyprus**, **Egypt** and **Pompeii** who first made extensive use of herbs with distillation methods dating back 3,500 B.C. This wisdom sailed across the Mediterranean and evidently reached **Hippocrates,** who utilized aromatherapy to enhance massage techniques a few centuries before the coming of Christ. Somewhere in the midst of this knowledge transfer, China and India also started to employ herbal remedies, and Ayurvedic medicine embraced essential oils extensively.

As civilizations transferred world power, the essential oil techniques from Greece travelled to **Rome,** who favored aromatherapy and fragrances. After the fall of the Roman Empire, **Persia** picked up these healing techniques and perfected the essential oil distillation process.

Sadly, the **Dark Ages** brought with it a disdain for Hippocrates' holistic approach. However, because the Catholic Church viewed bathing as sin, high esteem was given to aromatics – which coincidently are also antibacterial – to keep foul odor at bay. Little did they know that their perfume was also helping stave off sickness and disease! During this era, it is believed that Monks continued the healing tradition of essential oils and secretly kept herbal medicine alive in the halls of their monasteries.

Unfortunately, folk medicine was viewed as "witchcraft," and many herbalists were either burned at the stake or persecuted. Thankfully, the **Renaissance** resurrected herbal medicine, and physicians such as Paracelsus challenged his medical colleagues with testimonials of successful treating life-threatening concerns like leprosy.

Modern Era

What we know as modern "aromatherapy" was not introduced formally until French chemist **Rene Maurice Gattefosse** first coined the phrase in 1937. Although he wasn't necessarily a natural health advocate, he became interested in essential oils after a 1910 accident where he badly burned his hand, and used the first available salve in his laboratory: a pure, undiluted lavender oil compound that not only immediately eased the pain, but healed his injury without infection or scar. Because of Gattefosse's work, **Dr. Jean Valet** used essential oils to treat injured soldiers in the second world war, and this led to **Marguerite Maury** being the first person to "individually prescribe" essential oil combinations using a Tibetan technique for back massage that treated nerve endings along the spine. Since then, essential oils have become a staple in alternative medicine across the world. (1)

The Most Powerful Essential Oils

The list is long, but after careful research I've narrowed the top 10 essential oils for healing.

1. Clove (*Eugenia caryophyllata*) – Clove essential oil is commonly used as an antiseptic for oral infections and to kill a wide spectrum of microbes to keep disease at bay. To evaluate the effectiveness clove has as an antimicrobial agent, researchers from the University of Buenos Aires, Argentina, took a look at which bacteria are most sensitive to clove's potency. According to their study, clove has the greatest anti-microbial ability over *E. coli* and also exerted considerable control over *Staph aureus* and *Pseudomonas aeruginosa,* two bacteria that oftentimes lead to pneumonia and skin infections. (2)

2. Eucalyptus (*Eucalyptus Globulus*) – Used copiously by the Aborigines for most maladies in their villages, eucalyptus is a potent antibacterial, antispasmodic, and antiviral agent. Like clove essential oil, eucalyptus has a profound effect over *Staph* infections. Quite amazingly, recent research from VIT University in India showed (real-time) that when *Staph aureus* comes into contact with eucalyptus oil, the deadly bacterial completely lost viability within just 15 minutes of interaction! (3)

3. Frankincense (*Boswellia Carteri*) – Overshadowed the past several hundred years by its role in the "Christmas Story," frankincense is finally getting the attention it deserves as one of the most viable healing agents on the planet. The journal *Oncology Letters* published an article late last year that highlights the ability of this Biblical tree to kill cancer cells; specifically the MCF-7 and HS-1 cell lines, which cause breast and other tumors. (4) The essential oil has also been used with much success to treat issues related to digestion, the immune system, oral health, respiratory concerns and stress/anxiety.

4. Lavender (*Lavandula Angustifolia*) – Well-known for its soothing, calming properties, lavender is wonderful for accelerating healing time for burns, cuts, stings, and other wounds. It is jam-packed with antioxidant power, which is why researchers from Tunisia evaluated its ability to treat diabetes and oxidative stress in rats. Published in the journal *Lipids in Health and Disease*, the article tells us that lavender essential oils "significantly protected against the increase of blood glucose as well as the decrease of antioxidant enzyme activities." Ultimately, scientists discovered that lavender essential oil treatment helped induce a decrease in oxidative stress, which is known to cause heart disease and a slew of other health concerns, as well as increase antioxidant enzyme activities. (5)

Can this be the new diabetes and heart disease treatment? Maybe, maybe not. Either way, it'll be fun to watch the research come out on this topic!

5. Lemon (*Citrus limon*) – Various citrus essential oils are widely used to stimulate lymph drainage, to rejuvenate sluggish, dull skin and as a bug repellant. Lemon oil stands out, however, as research has recently discovered that it carries useful antimicrobial and anti-inflammatory properties. (6) Lemon, along with a number of other widely used oils, is now being praised for its ability to combat food-born pathogens! (7)

6. Oregano (*Origanum vulgare*) – Several research studies have demonstrated the improving effect on performance, changes in blood count, antibacterial, antifungal and immunomodulating abilities of oregano oil. It's actually quite amazing – the health benefits of oregano seem limitless. To give you a sample of its wide-spread potency, WebMD reports,

Oregano is used for respiratory tract disorders such as coughs, asthma, croup, and bronchitis. It is also used for gastrointestinal (GI) disorders such as heartburn and bloating. Other uses include treating menstrual cramps, rheumatoid arthritis, urinary tract disorders including urinary tract infections (UTIs), headaches, and heart conditions. The oil of oregano is taken by mouth for intestinal parasites, allergies, sinus pain, arthritis, cold and flu, swine flu, earaches, and fatigue. It is applied to the skin for skin conditions including acne, athlete's foot, oily skin, dandruff, canker sores, warts, ringworm, rosacea, and psoriasis; as well as for insect and spider bites, gum disease, toothaches, muscle pain, and varicose veins. Oregano oil is also used topically as an insect repellent. (8)

7. Peppermint (*Mentha Piperita*) – Pleasantly suitable for an abundance of oral and topical uses, peppermint may be the most versatile essential oil in the world. Literally, there are few issues that it can't help. Possibly the most fascinating aspect of peppermint is that recent research suggests that it is literally *antibiotic resistant*. According to an article published in the journal *Phytomedicine* in 2013, "Reduced usage of antibiotics could be employed as a treatment strategy to decrease the adverse effects and possibly to reverse the beta-lactam antibiotic resistance," due to the powerful effects of peppermint oil. (9)

This is absolutely groundbreaking because antibiotic-resistant bacteria have been a major cause of concern for many Americans who are simply ruining their health by taking too many of these dangerous drugs. Can you imagine a world where your doctor prescribes peppermint essential oil for the common cold and flu instead of antibiotics? We can! And we hope that more research like this reaches mainstream media to get the word out!

8. Rosemary (*Rosmarinus officinalis*) – One amazing healing effect of rosemary that many people are unaware of is its ability to normalize blood pressure. Used for centuries to improve everything from memory and brain function to relieving common aches and pains, rosemary even has a history of stimulating hair growth. But most people don't think of rosemary mimicking their blood pressure pills!

In one of the few human studies evaluating this phenomenon, researchers from the Universidad Complutense de Madrid took 32 hypotensive patients and measured how their dangerously low blood pressure fared under rosemary essential oil treatments for 72 weeks. The results? Simply astounding! In addition to observing that rosemary could raise blood pressure to normal limits in a vast majority of the volunteers, it was discovered that overall mental and physical quality of life was drastically improved, which highlights the far-reaching healing effects that this ancient oil has on health and wellness. (10)

9. Sandalwood (*Santalum album*) – Oftentimes used to soothe and heal sore throats, sandalwood is a gentle bactericide that is more potent than most give it credit for. According to research published last year, sandalwood essential oil also has an uncanny ability to inhibit both tyrosinase and cholinesterase, which affects several physiological processes from melanin production to proper nervous system function. The results were so significant that scientists concluded that, "There is a great potential of this essential oil for use in the treatment of Alzheimer's disease!" ([11](#))

10. Tea Tree (*Melaleuca alternifolia*) – Last, but certainly not least, tea tree is a wound healer with a rich history of use as a local antiseptic for burns and cuts as well to treat a wide spectrum of bacterial and fungal infections (including athletes foot and jock itch). Known in the science community as "volatile" because of its sheer power in killing microbes, a study was actually conducted to determine whether it could be damage your DNA. Don't worry, thousands of years of use wasn't done in vain. According to the study published in *The Journal of Ethnopharmacology*, researchers finally put this criticism to rest last year by proving that tea tree oil is not toxic and is completely safe for use. ([12](#))

The way I see it, if an essential oil is so powerful that scientists need to test if it can cause damage to your genes, it has got to be doing something that is turning heads! And it's not just tea tree oil. All of these oils are super-healers and should be in medicine cabinets all over the world.

Uses & Applications

Because they are so potent, you must also dilute essential oils in one way or another. The following are some common ways to use them appropriately:

- **Baths:** 10 drops mixed with 1 cup of salt makes a fantastic aromatherapy for circulatory, muscular, respiratory, skin and sleep problems in addition to calming your nerves. Generally, it is advisable to avoid potent oils that could irritate the skin such as lemon, oregano or tea tree; instead, use soothing oils like eucalyptus, lavender, and sandalwood.
- **Compresses:** 5 drops per 4 oz. of water. Soak cloth and apply for bruises, infections, aches and pains.
- **Inhalations:** 5 drops in a diffuser or in hot water for sinus or headache relief.
- **Salves:** A 2.5% dilution is recommended, which is 10 drops per 1 ounce of oil, for relaxation and to alleviate joint/muscle soreness.

Clary Sage

The medicinal use of clary sage dates back to the age of Rome and Greece. Officially named *Salvia sclarea,* it was used for eye conditions, to clear (*clar*ify) the eyes, potentially with the mucilaginous seeds. In 1653, Dante Culpeper's work *Complete Herbal* described clary sage as such:

"The seed put into the eyes clears them from motes, and such like things gotten within the lids to offend them, as also clears them from white and red spots on them. The mucilage of the seed made with water, and applied to **tumours***, or swellings, disperses and takes them away; as also draws forth splinters, thorns, or other* **things gotten into the flesh***. The leaves used with vinegar, either by itself, or with a little honey, doth help* **boils, felons, and the hot inflammation** *that are gathered by their pains, if applied before it be grown too great… The juice of the herb put into ale or beer, and drank, brings down* **women's courses***, and expels the after-birth."(1)*

Centuries later, we still use clary sage in similar ways, particularly for its anti-inflammatory benefits and role in women's health.

What is Clary Sage?

Primarily originating from the Mediterranean region, clary sage is a *Salvia* variant, which you may know from your ornamental perennial garden or from its cousin *sage*, which is used for both culinary and medicinal purposes. Salvia are part of the larger *Lamiaceae* distinction, the mint family, which is full of fragrant plants rich in essential oil and healing qualities.

Clary sage is used in both herb and essential oil form, and even the seeds have nutritional value. As with any herb or essential oil, where clary sage is grown, how and when it is harvested, and the parts of the plant used all play a part in the quality and components. (2)

Covered in spikes of flowers, fragrant, and grown as a perennial, it's little wonder that the ancients found use for this favorite family of herbs!

Composition of Clary Sage

Clary sage essential oil is derived from the flowering tops and contains many components known for their anti-inflammatory and calming benefits, including linalool (a major component of lavender essential oil), linalyl acetate (excellent for anti-inflammatory benefits on skin), and a component called sclareol. The method of extraction may affect the components found in the essential oil, so always be aware of your source before using an oil therapeutically. (3)

Aside from anti-inflammatory abilities, clary sage is also known to be relaxing and antidepressant, antifungal, and antimicrobial. It is also an excellent antioxidant source, with a large portion of its composition coming from caryophyllene oxide, a powerful antioxidant that may even be implicated in fighting the effects of aging and prolonging life! (4, 5)

Another component, sclareol, has shown some promising things in lab tests. Over the last couple of decades but as recently as this year (2015), studies have emerged that analyze sclareol's effect on cancer cells. With the caveat that these benefits occurred within the confines of lab cultures and dose adjustments, sclareol may have an impact on the way that cancer cells proliferate, and it could help induce apoptosis (cancer cell death). (6, 7)

While this does not tell us how much potential sclareol has to directly treat cancer – and it's exciting to think about where that could go one day! – it is a common thread that we see in many antioxidant-rich essential oils. This is especially interesting for clary sage, which also contains esters. Esters are commonly avoided in those who have cancer, as the phytoestrogen ability can, in theory, feed into cancer. With potential anti-cancer benefits built into clary sage, you have to wonder if it is meant to work as a whole package that ultimately delivers only benefits!

How to Use Clary Sage

Really, you can't go wrong with antioxidants and anti-inflammatory effects. There are a few uses that stand out as particularly effective for clary sage, though, with plenty of research to back them up.

Antimicrobial skin protection — In 2015, researchers in Poland published results of their search for effective treatments for antibiotic resistant bacteria. When applied to resistant strains of the *Staphylococcus* bacteria, clary sage was able to kill the bacteria, where other antibiotics failed. ([8](#))

Earlier, in 2012, a blend of essential oils was tested against *Staphylococcus* bacteria, as well as *E. coli* and the pervasive Candida fungus. A blend of lavender, clary sage, and ylang ylang was found to be synergistically effective against all three. ([9](#))

Stress Relief — Aromatherapy is linked with relaxation and stress-relief in many of our minds, even before we become familiar with essential oils. I know that's all I knew of them at first! But certain oils are more effective than others, and clary stage stands out. In fact, when a group of essential oils were tested for antidepressant abilities, clary sage showed far and away the most potential, indicating it as a potential stand-alone treatment thanks to dopamine regulation. ([10](#))

Women's Health — Clary sage is most commonly known as an herb and essential oil for women's health issues, thanks to its esters and phytoestrogen ability, exhibiting benefits in all phases of life. Young women dealing with menstrual pain have found relief, even moreso than what acetaminophen could provide. ([11](#)) Women with dysmenorrhea found similar relief. ([12](#))

In childbirth, where pain is often exacerbated by anxiety and stress, clary sage and chamomile exhibit strong pain relieving results in a safe, easily administered manner. In fact, when a midwifery practice implemented the use of these oils both topically in a carrier oil and via diffusion, the use of pain relieving opioids begain to decrease significantly. (13)

Finally, as women reach menopausal years, the use of antidepressants begins to increase dramatically. Clary sage may help to ease this stressful transition of life, reducing cortisol levels and exhibiting and antidepressant-like effect (14)

For maximum effects, try blending clary sage with oils that have similar properties, like lavender and chamomile.

Clove

Just as its parent plant is evergreen, thriving in every season, clove essential oil is strong and adaptable. Clove's first form is the handpicked flower buds of the *Eugenia caryophyllata* of the Maluku Islands in Indonesia. Each bud is picked by hand, then dried until the pink blossoms have turned brown. From there, the dried cloves are ground and used in cooking or distilled for their essential oil content.

For two millennia, clove has been used for fragrance and spice, making international interest a couple hundred years after the Chinese first documented use. Because of clove's **eugenol** properties, the essential oil in particular has found use in alternative wellness remedies.

Clove's nutritional profile is impressive, as well. They are a good source of vitamin K, fiber, iron, magnesium, and calcium. Most impressively, two teaspoons of clove boast over 120% of our daily need for manganese, a mineral that is implicated in the prevention of osteoporosis, anemia, and premenstrual syndrome (PMS). (1)

Antioxidant Power — More and more, researchers are discovering just how powerful antioxidants are and how important they are for health. The National Institute on Aging developed a way for us to quantify antioxidant capability in the Oxygen Radical Absorbance Capacity (ORAC) system of measurement. Within the ORAC system, cloves come in as one of the highest valued antioxidants, towering over sorghum, the next on the list, by a difference of more than 50,000. (2) As a concentrated essential oil, there is simply no comparison. However, some sources claim the following:

Essential Oil Antioxidant Capacity		Foods Antioxidant Capacity	
Clove	1,078,700	Vitamin E oil	3,309
Myrrh	379,800	Pomegranates	3,037
Coriander	298,300	Blueberries	2,400
Fennel	238,400	Kale	1,770
Clary sage	221,000	XanGo juice	1,644
Marjoram	130,900	Tahitian Noni	1,506
Melissa	134,300	Strawberries	1,540
Ylang ylang	130,000	Spinach	1,260
Wintergreen	101,800	Raspberries	1,220
Geranium	101,000	Brussels sprouts	980
Ginger	99,300	Plums	949
Black Pepper	79,700	Broccoli florets	890
Vetiver	74,300	Beets	840
Basil	54,000	Oranges	750
Patchouli	49,400	Red grapes	739
White fir	47,900	Red bell peppers	710
Peppermint	37,300	Cherries	670
Dill	35,600	Yellow corn	400
Lime	26,200	Eggplant	390
Cypress	24,300	Limu juice	305
Grapefruit	22,600	Carrots	210
Thyme	15,960		
Oregano	15,300	**Essential Oils Antioxidant Capacity**	
Cassia	14,800	Frankincense	630
Cinnamon bark	7,100	Spearmint	540
Wild Orange	1,890	Lavender	360
Lemongrass	1,780	Rosemary	330
Helichrysum	1,740	Roman chamomile	240
Lemon	660	Sandalwood	160

Disclaimer: *once hosted by the USDA website*, a peer-reviewed table of ORAC valued peer-reviewed resources is not available. The above chart is from *BioSource Naturals*.

A Note about ORAC Value

While the ins and outs of free radicals and antioxidants aren't necessary to commit to memory, it's important to acknowledge the healing power that antioxidants carry and to become familiar with antioxidant levels in foods and substances. The stronger the antioxidant level, the more you want to utilize that food, spice, or essential oil.

To break antioxidants down to a basic level, they are, on a molecular level, able to target and eliminate free radicals, then reverse the damage that has been done.

Free radicals are also molecules, but they set in motion a cascade of cellular problems that can lead to cell death and even cancer.

The cellular-level repair that antioxidants are able to accomplish is well-studied, with research connecting it to slowed aging and inhibited disease processes.

In short, antioxidants are a wellspring of healing, and clove essential oil is the tap!

Common Uses

With all of that antioxidant healing power, you probably already have a feel for the potential that clove essential oil (CEO) carries. With great power comes great responsibility, though, and CEO carries as much potential for damage as it does for healing.

A recent study, published in the *Journal of Immunotoxicology,* demonstrates this balance between effectiveness and caution. After investigating the effects of eugenol – CEO's most prominent property – on the liver, they discovered two sides of one coin. Eugenol in low doses protected the liver, not only against at least one cause of liver disease but also against inflammation and cell death. On the other hand, "a larger dose amplifies the liver injury via oxidant and inflammatory effects." (3)

This is both good news and a warning, that:

1. CEO is a powerful substance.
2. Powerful substances should be handled carefully, under the guidance of knowledge, wisdom, and common sense.

With this caution in mind, we can explore the benefits of CEO when used safely and appropriately – and there are many benefits!

We've already seen its anti-inflammatory capability, and with inflammatory illness so heavily plaguing our society, you can imagine the implications that has. There are other effects of eugenol that make CEO beneficial for disease prevention and oral health. Let's explore just a few of these properties in light of current research.

Antibacterial – Clove essential oil is widely understood to be generally antibacterial, but the University of Buenos Aires took the time to pinpoint bacteria that clove was especially able to target. They found that *E. coli* was particularly susceptible to CEO, followed by *Staph aureus* and *Pseudomonas aeruginosa*. With all of these connected to significant illness, skin infections, and pneumonia, CEO is a valuable tool for disease prevention. (4)

Antifungal – Candida is a devastating, pervasive problem in our culture, and one that remains a personal soapbox of mine. Our diets high in sugar and acidification kill beneficial gut microbes and colonize Candida. In mainstream medicine, nystatin is used to manage yeast infections, though it never addresses the root causes and can bring side effects of its own. Published in the journal *Oral Microbiology & Immunology,* researchers weighed the effects of clove essential oil against nystatin, finding it just as effective, but as a natural substance rather than chemical concoction. (5)

Analgesic and Antiseptic – Clove essential oil is a longtime dental remedy, dating back to 1640 in French documentation "Practice of Physic," and beyond in Chinese tradition. To this day, clove remains a go-to for dental needs.

The *Journal of Dentistry* published a comparison between CEO in a gel and benzocaine, the topical numbing agent the precedes needles in dentistry. In over seventy participants, no difference was recorded between benzocaine and CEO gel, indicating the same numbing effects. (6)

Aside from pain relief and numbing, CEO's dental benefits extend to slowed decay and remineralization. Underscoring this point, the Indian Department of Public Health Dentistry conducted a controlled study to evaluate clove essential oil, its lead molecules, and fluoride against decay caused by apple juice. CEO emerged as a promising mineralization tool, "significantly" decreasing decalcification, and actually remineralizing teeth. (7)

As a side note, I find it interesting that fluoride is so heavily used and recommended when there are clear, natural alternatives. It's one more reason to immerse ourselves in the ancient wisdom of natural health and remedies!

Recommendation: For antioxidant and immune support, add 1 drop of clove essential oil to a tsp of honey, maple syrup, or coconut oil and wash down with some water. Pair with a drop of orange and/or cinnamon to further the benefits.

Eucalyptus

Migrating all the way from Down Under to China, the current top producer, eucalyptus essential oil comes from the Austrailian-native Tasmanium Blue Gum tree, an evergreen with a relatively recent medicinal history. Upon first Western discovery, eucalyptus was dubbed "Sidney Peppermint" thanks to similarities to the English *Mentha piperita*. Current uses do indicate similarities between the two, but we know now as they quickly realized then, that eucalyptus stands out as a strong, efficient oil in its own right.

Eucalyptus' Secret Weapon

Essential oils can carry hundreds of components in every drop, each with its own benefits and effects. Chemists analyze these components to determine what the oil is doing and how, which helps us to know how to use the oils safely and effectively.

At first, the strong component in eucalyptus was named "eucalyptol," indicating its uniqueness among other oils. Now, we call it *cineole*, and its effects and potential are quite remarkable. Scientists can't get enough of this powerful substance, with over a thousand studies returned on a search for *cineole,* and more added all the time.

Eucalyptus introduced us to cineole, with 80-95% of eucalyptus essential oil comprised of it, but scientists have since discovered that other plants can carry it as well. Some notable essential oils that contain cineole include ginger, helichrysum, rosemary, tea tree, and peppermint – so, perhaps the initial association between eucalyptus and peppermint was not so far off base! In fact, the similarities shared between plants and their essential oil derivatives may contribute to that amazing, mysterious synergistic effect that essential oil blends create.

Looking to the Research

With so much research directed toward cineole and eucalyptus, there is much to say about studies done on its effects and the possible implications of their results.

Eucalyptus essential oil is proving itself as a strong respiratory support, with anti-inflammatory effects and benefits for breathing. Not only do we enjoy it for acute respiratory symptoms, but a breakthrough study published in *Drug Research* looked even further – intro chronic illness. This study evaluated the effect of inhaled eucalyptus essential oil in patients with Chronic Obstructive Pulmonary Disease (COPD) and found it beneficial for long-term treatment with promising results. (1)

Another impressive find relates to the antibacterial effects of eucalyptus essential oil. Drug-resistant bacteria are a major public health concern worldwide, with both treatment and prevention desperately needed. So, researchers at the University of Illinois looked to eucalyptus for an answer that,

"...responds to the need to reduce the number of contagious MDR/ XRD-TB patients, protect their immediate environment, and

interrupt the rapid spread by laying the groundwork for an inhalation therapy based on anti-TB-active constituents of the essential oil (EO) of Eucalyptus citriodora."

By analyzing the reactions between eucalyptus and the resistant tuberculosis (TB) bacteria, they found that some variations of the oil successfully killed the bacteria more than 90% of the time. (2)

On what seems to be a completely different note, French scientists shared their findings with the *Journal of Food Science* after evaluating six different oils with antioxidant status for their ability to address hypertension. (3) The efficacy of eucalyptus oil on heart relaxation was significant, and while we cannot say that means you can neglect antihypertensive medications, the research is promising and we hope to see further details emerge over time.

History of Eucalyptus

Folklore and oral history may not be as solid as scientific evidence, but they tell a story that is worth acknowledging.

The story goes that an English settler in Australia badly wounded his thumb with an axe. His father, who knew Aboriginal remedies, suggested tying a eucalyptus leaf to the thumb like a tight bandage once it had been stitched closed. This remedy was known as "kino," and was used frequently. The settler's surgeon later commented on how well his thumb had healed without succumbing to infection. With this and similar stories circulating, Joseph Bosisto and other pharmacists saw the opportunity to begin producing eucalyptus essential oil commercially, which they did in 1852.

Varied and Unique Benefits

In the light of popular use, to excuse the pun, towns used eucalyptus oil that was converted into a gas to light their homes, hotels, and shops. Little did they know that they stumbled upon some pretty powerful aromatherapy benefits as well!

While we don't light our homes with eucalyptus, we have tried a few of these unique and effective remedies including the potent oil:

- **Expectorant and Purifier** – When you've got a cold or the flu, you might feel like your head will explode if it cannot expel mucous. Eucalyptus works as an expectorant to ease that discomfort, and as a bonus, it can help the body to remove toxins and threats that make it all feel worse. Try dropping several drops of eucalyptus essential oil into a diffuser while you sleep to help clear your breathing and improve sleep. Or, for a more powerful application, drop 10 drops into hot water, then lean over it with a towel "tented" around your head. Breathe deeply for five to ten minutes and enjoy the relief.
- **Scalp Tonic** – Cleanse and refresh your scalp and hair with a few drops of eucalyptus mixed into coconut or olive oil. The carriers will moisturize while the eucalyptus relieves itchy skin and dandruff.
- **Hands & Feet Cleanser** – Grease can't stand a chance against eucalyptus, making a strong case for its inclusion in homemade cleansers – or, if you're up for a real treat, a refreshing salt soak for hands or feet.

- **Potent Cleaning Agent** – If you enjoy the fragrance of eucalyptus, you may already include it in your cleaning recipes. What you may not know is that it is highly antimicrobial, helping to clear surfaces of potential illness. If you're making a cleaner of any sort, you need to add eucalyptus.
- **Essential Filters** – Spread the love! Eucalyptus dropped onto the air filer in your home can help to circulate fresh, rejuvenating scents to the whole house.
- **Stain Removal** – If you have stained fabric surfaces, give eucalyptus essential oil a try at removal. Of course, you want to make sure (in an inconspicuous spot) that the oil is compatible with the blend of fabric you have – just in case a random synthetic blend reacts poorly to the eucalyptus oil.
- **Air Freshener** – Refresh the mind and lift the spirits with a spritz bottle? With ten drops of eucalyptus EO added to a small spritzer bottle filled with distilled water after a long day at work, you can make this happen. Simply spray 12 inches from your face and enjoy inhaling the gentle mist.
- **Odor Control** – After a long day of summer play, the summer laundry room can become quite noxious. Run stinky clothes and shoes through the dryer with a rag soaked in water and a few drops of eucalyptus essential oil. For shoes, stick the rag down into the shoe. This can help prevent odors as well as help keep the shape intact!
- **Pets** – Yes, even Fido can enjoy the benefits of eucalyptus oil. In fact, centuries of use suggest that eucalyptus is safe in nearly any application, as long as common sense is followed. Keep it out of eyes and wounds (both yours and your pet's!) for safety, and always dilute properly.

Frankincense

Tradition tells us that, in Babylon, nearly 60,000 pounds of frankincense burned annually for its aromatics and its role in rituals. Later, we see the Magi bringing frankincense along with gold and myrrh to the infant Jesus. More than a costly, fragrant gift, the ancient healing benefits of frankincense are well documented and have made this tree resin famous today.

Ayurvedic medicine, in practice for centuries, uses frankincense (referred to as "dhoop" and it use as "dhoopan") for wound healing, female hormonal issues, arthritis, and air purification. In many cultures – including Somali, Ethiopian, Arabian, and Indian – frankincense has daily uses. Burning it in the house is said to bring good health, and burning it in the evening is meant to purify the home and the residents' clothing. (1)

Properties of Frankincense

Frankincense (Boswellia carterii, Boswellia serrata, and the other Boswellia species), as with all plants and their essential oils, carries many different molecules with different purposes. Some stand out as prominent in certain substances, as is the case with boswellic acids (BAs) in frankincense. Although there is some debate whether or not BA is too large a compound to survive conventional essential oil filtration systems, there are studies in the literature that claim they are indeed part of frankincense oil (2)

Nonetheless, the healing benefits of frankincense have traditionally centered on disease prevention and anti-inflammatory properties, and researchers have been able to confirm that boswellic acids contain a potent ability to modify the immune system as well. (3) Part of having a more efficient immune system is the regulation of inflammation, as well, which can have effects topically or systemically. (4)

Another promising property is the proposed frankincense cancer cure that we've read so much about in the past few years. In several studies, frankincense has demonstrated anti-cancer properties and the ability to mitigate many different kinds of cancer cells. (5) As more studies are conducted, the implications of this ability will be exciting to watch unfold!

The jury is still out as to the exact mechanism(s) explaining why frankincense essential oil is so beneficial to cancer patients. However, advances in recent research suggest that Beta-elemene – a cancer fighting terpene found in frankincense and myrrh with the ability to cross the blood brain barrier – may be partly responsible. As stated by the Memorial Sloan Kettering Cancer Center,

"Beta-elemene is a compound found in plants such as celery, mint, and in many others used in traditional medicine. Although the pure form is not used as dietary supplement, some cancer patients use herbs high in beta-elemene as treatment. Beta-elemene was shown to prevent growth of cancer cells in laboratory cells by different mechanisms. A few poorly designed studies done in humans showed that it may improve quality of life in cancer patients. It is unclear if raw herbs containing beta-elemene have the same effects in humans. More research is needed." (6)

Some even suggest that the amount of β-elemene that frankincense and myrrh contain could very well explain why so many people claim that both oils have been instrumental to them beating cancer God's way. (7)

At the end of the day, once we know the basic properties of an herb, root and resin we are able to determine the best ways to utilize it.

Let's take a closer look at what the components of frankincense mean for our daily lives...

1. Boosting the Immune System

The immune system is intricate and amazing, interacting with every system of the body to prevent and fight disease. One of the primary mechanisms of the immune system is the influx of white blood cells, or lymphocytes, the main defense method that the body has. Inflammation is another component of the immune system, but in an unhealthy body, it goes overboard and becomes problematic.

By studying the way that frankincense affects the immune system in mice, we have an idea of its interaction with our own immune response. In Phytotherapy Research, the results of this study were noted to include:

- Cytokine production
- Slowed hypersensitivity
- Increased immunoglobins
- Improved T-cell interactions

The bottom line is that multiple areas of the immune system are regulated under the influence of frankincense. (8)

2. Fighting Pain and Inflammation

The beauty of immunomodulators is that they can stimulate an under-productive immune system that allows illness to creep in, while also relaxing an over-productive immune system that attacks itself or benign substances with inflammation, often becoming painful, chronic, and debilitating.

By regulating inflammation, frankincense oil is a powerful tool not only for acute illness but for chronic and autoimmune disorders such as Crohn's disease, rheumatoid arthritis, ulcerative colitis, and bronchial asthma. (9) Weight and other metabolic issues are tied to inflammation as well, so even when these chronic conditions are not an issue, inflammatory illness is still a concern to monitor and prevent.

While inflammatory conditions are often painful, frankincense can help with other pain relief as well. In Omani culture, it is traditionally used for pain in muscles, intestinal discomfort, and arthritic pain. (10)

In 2014, researchers local to Oman tested frankincense essential oil and extracts to validate this practice compared with aspirin. Of the various preparations tested, frankincense oil showed the strongest pain inhibiting results with over 50% in both early and late phase pain. Researchers concluded that,

"The present study provided the scientific justification about the analgesic properties of the essential oils, extract, and various sub-fractions obtained from the resin of B. sacra, thus validating its use in traditional folk medicines and other products; and hence supporting the development in the analgesic properties of bioactive natural substances." (11)

3. Preventing & Treating Cancer

While we do know that the various forms of frankincense (essential oils, extracts, pure resin, etc.) the potential to fight cancer, much is left to be understood, making this a controversial topic in the natural health and research world.

Current research demonstrates anti-mutagenic and apoptotic (prevents cell death) abilities. Though the results have occurred in lab tests and we have yet to see how to best replicate these results in active cancer in humans, the demonstrated results remain. Researchers found that boswellic acids are "cytotoxic to ovarian cancer cells at pharmacologically achievable concentrations" and "may form the basis of a novel anticancer treatment for ovarian cancer, perhaps alongside conventional chemotherapy." (12) Studies continue to emerge, demonstrating similar effects on bladder (13), breast (14), colon (15), skin (16), stomach (17), and pancreatic cancers. (18)

For those who have added frankincense to their cancer care plan, the benefits may go beyond anti-tumor effects. Conventional treatment is often still required, but can be more painful and difficult than the symptoms of cancer itself. Brain cancer patients, for example, sometimes experience swelling in the head called cerebral edema after their tumors have been removed. Steroid treatment is common but also associated with difficult side effects and complications.

Frankincense, on the other hand, has shown remarkable effects against this particular problem. In 2011, a clinical trial evaluating 44 individuals monitored frankincense as a remedy for cerebral edema. In 60% of the patients, the swelling was reduced by 75% or more. The concluding remarks called for frankincense to be prescribed for cerebral edema in these circumstances, avoiding the struggles of steroid therapy. (19)

For a similar call for a shift in treatment protocol, much more research must be done. Unfortunately, because cancer is such a deadly disease with a limited opportunity to administer effective treatments, testing the efficacy of alternative treatments, administering control studies, and adjusting administration and dosage all pose ethical roadblocks. So while specific answers may come slowly, it's plain to see that the potential and properties exist. With little to no side effects associated with frankincense essential oil, we have little to lose and much to gain when adding it to our daily routines or pairing it with cancer protocols in conjunction with an oncological approach.

Recommendations: In spite of the frankincense oil cancer cure controversy, the powerful role that frankincense plays in immunity, inflammatory control, pain relief, and anti-cancer potential makes it a necessary supplement to have around the house "just in case." Vaporizors, salves, supplementation and diffusion are all beneficial ways to use it.

Some effective personal uses are to:

- Mix 1 drop of frankincense per 2 drops of carrier oil of your choice, and apply over the tumor directly.
- Take 1 drop of frankincense with 4 ounces of water first thing in the morning and right before bed, or mix with 1/2 tsp honey, maple syrup, or coconut oil.
- Put 1 drop into a gel capsule and take with food.

Helichrysum

A beautiful annual flower, helichrysum is from the daisy family, named for its appearance – not unlike a burst of sunshine! *Helichrysum* is actually a whole species, with many varieties beneath it. Many are cultivated in the US for their ornamental beauty, but they are native to the Mediterranean region. Other helichrysum are from as far south as South Africa, and as well-established as to be part of traditional medicine in that region, as well. (1)

In historical terms, helichrysum has been selected for centuries, sometimes indicated as a gift to the Greek gods in the form of dried flowerheads. Now, it is more aptly considered a gift to us, with age-reversing capabilities and healing factors packaged in a delightful, bright flower.

All About Helichrysum

When it wasn't being offered to the residents of Mount Olympus, helichrysum had traditional applications for a number of conditions. Respiratory ailments, skin trouble, live and gall bladder issues, inflammation, insomnia, and infections all came with a "prescription" for helichrysum. Not all of these uses have been confirmed yet, but one by one the scientific community is discovering that the ancients were wise when it came to their choice in remedy.

Helichrysum italica and *H. angustifolia* are the interchangeable names for the commonly used essential oil, though we can look at the whole species when gaining an understanding of the general components it carries. Within the essential oil, flavonoids, ketones, and terpenes exhibit strong effects, and while these components are typically indicators that caution should be used, helichrysum is an incredibly safe and versatile oil in terms of application. (2)

The effects that have been researched are convincing, and it's no wonder that helichrysum is also called "immortelle" – the fountain of youth was an antioxidant-rich, essential-oil filled flower all along!

Benefits of Helichrysum Essential Oil

The older the herb and essential oil, the more we have to discover. From generation to generation, ancient wisdom was passed along and honed, creating a cultural understanding of medicinal properties of local plants. Many factors have changed that dynamic, simultaneously leading us to information in other regions and losing some of the wisdom we might have had in our own culture. As scientists dig into the effects and benefits of these substances of old, one by one, we are finding confirmation time and again that traditional remedies are often traceable in science.

Here are some of the traditionally-held uses of helichrysum, and the helichrysum essential oil preparation in particular, that are finding traction in modern research:

- **Antibiotic Resistance Solution** — Antimicrobial substances have been used for centuries, but the rise of modern antibiotics and subsequent overuse has created drug-resistant superbugs. Now, natural products are regaining the spotlight as effective treatments. In 2009, French scientists evaluated helichrysum essential oil as a potential natural antibiotic, and they were not disappointed. They noted that helichrysm essential oil (*H. italicum*, to be specific), "significantly reduces the multidrug resistance" of multiple bacteria. (3) This is a potentially lifesaving ability, potentiating antibiotic treatments when they are needed most.

- **Antimicrobial activity** — In its native regions, helichrysum is known as anti-inflammatory, and antimicrobial. To begin to explore the validity of these claims, Iranian researchers tested the composition of helichrysum essential oil on both Gram negative and Gram positive bacteria, as well as fungal contaminants. The team concluded not only a moderate effect on both kinds of bacteria, but that helichrysum essential oil "had a substantial fungicidal effect on the fungi under study." (4)

- **Stress & Burnout Relief** — As part of a 2013 article in the *Journal for Alternative and Complementary Medicine*, helichrysum essential oil was blended with peppermint and basil oils to form a potentially relaxing blend. Individuals participated in a double blind, randomized, placebo study to determine whether aromatherapy actually exhibits relaxing effects. The individuals in the study described themselves as dealing with burnout and mental exhaustion. Since taking the time to take care of ourselves is a big part of reducing fatigue and stress, both the placebo and oils reduced the fatigue somewhat. However, the essential oil blend was much greater, confirming their ability to truly affect our brain and body systems, beyond placebo or general self-care effects. (5)

- **Anti-Inflammatory** — When the immune system's normal functions go into overdrive, painful and sometimes life threatening inflammation can set in anywhere from skin conditions to arthritis to heart disease. That places anti-inflammatory substances as one of the most important remedies and health boosters we can get our hands on. Helichrysum essential oil falls into that category, displaying anti-inflammatory effects in a 2004 article in the *Journal of Ethnopharmacology*. (6)

Where Helichrysum Shines

As exciting as these remedies and benefits are, helichrysum's near legendary effects are found in its anti-aging capabilities. As I mentioned, it is sometimes known as ***immortelle* or *everlasting***, demonstrating the folk knowledge that it may be a secret to aging well – or perhaps reversing the toll that age has already taken!

Anti-aging is more than another candle added to the cake – it's a whole process, and any process can be slowed or reversed, regardless of what the calendar says. The key, almost undoubtedly, lies in the combination of anti-inflammatory and antioxidant capabilities of the plant and oil, with helichrysum being found as one of seventeen essential oils that remain highly active antioxidants even at lower concentrations. (7)

Oxidative stress is a major component of aging, which is a primary risk factor for heart disease. The very definition of oxidative stress is cellular breakdown, with free radicals wreaking havoc on tissues – hence the loss of collagen, stiffness and aches and pains, and so on.

When the body can produce enough antioxidants and is supported via dietary and supplemental antioxidants, not only is the breakdown stopped in its tracks, but the cells themselves can actually be repaired and restored.

Helichrysum as a whole herb remedy is one such antioxidant, and the essential oil blends stress relieving ability with antioxidant capability and anti-inflammatory strength to provide just what the skin needs to begin to repair years of damage.

Recommendation:

Include helichrysum essential oil in topical blends as well as with Epsom salt for relaxing aromatic baths that address all stress, aging, and skincare all at once.

Lavender

For over 2,500 years, lavender has been documented in medicinal and religious uses, from ancient texts through modern movements. Beginning with Egyptian mummification, lavender moved to Roman bathhouses, fragrance, and cooking. Later, it's possible that Mary anointed Jesus' feet with it, given the Greek name *naardus,* listed Biblically as nard or spikenard:

"Mary then took a pound of very costly perfume of pure nard, and anointed the feet of Jesus and wiped His feet with her hair; and the house was filled with the fragrance of the perfume."

~ John 12:3

In modern times, lavender is credited as the essential oil that Gattefosse instinctively covered his burned arm with, igniting a renewed interest in essential oils and inspiring the term *aromatherapy.* That lavender has stood the test of time, inspiring interest in so many eras, cultures, and generations, is a testament to the varied and effective capabilities it carries.

Lavender's Health Properties

While the millennia have used lavender based on tradition and ancient wisdom, modern science is only just now discovering the mechanisms of lavender's benefits and its rich health benefits. To scratch the surface of its capabilities, let's look at the top 5 properties that lavender essential oil brings to the table – a table riddled with health concerns.

Lavender is a Potent Antioxidant

A recurring theme in any natural health discussion, antioxidants are, in effect, the super healers that our culture needs. The free radicals created by toxins, pollutants, chemicals, and even stress are the culprits for a cascade of cellular damage, immune inhibition, and limitless health risks – including chronic illness and cancer.

If free radicals are the villain, antioxidants are the hero.

The body itself creates antioxidants in the form of the enzymes glutathione peroxidase (GSH-Px), superoxide dismutase (SOD) and catalase (CAT), among others. But we expose our bodies to an onslaught of free radicals and drain our bodies in sedentary lifestyles, so our natural production is not always sufficient.

We've already seen some super antioxidants, like clove essential oil, and lavender joins the ranks as a powerful natural antioxidant support. Not long ago, Chinese researchers observed that lavender essential oil would attenuate all three major antioxidant enzyme levels in mice within the first day of treatment. (1) In Romania, researchers noted similar activity using inhaled lavender for an hour each day – and this study also noted protection against the cell death (apoptosis) that can lead to severe illness and cancer. (2)

Lavender Can Help Manage Diabetes

Tunisian traditional medicine utilizes lavender, grown in their region, as a remedy and health support. In 2014, local scientists released the results of a study they had conducted to determine how this traditional remedy actually works. Their findings were fascinating.

The researchers established a 15-day study of diabetic rats, during which lavender essential oil was used as a treatment. The lavender treatment protected against all of the following, each one a hallmark of the diabetic illness:

* Blood glucose increases
* Metabolic illness
* Weight gain
* Depletion of antioxidants
* Liver and kidney disfunction and lipoperoxidation

The presence of unmitigated free radicals, the depletion of antioxidants and liver and kidney function, the descent into metabolic illness and weight gain – all are components of diabetes as an illness. Potent antioxidants like lavender essential oil are allies in the pursuit of long term health, and this study underscored its abilities. (3)

With more research and concrete answers, perhaps one day lavender essential oil and other natural treatments will be the standard for diabetic prevention and relief!

Lavender Protects Neurological Health

While Tunisian researchers were analyzing metabolic health, lavender was taking center stage in published neurological research, and for similar reasons – to confirm longstanding traditional use. Lavender has long been used for stress, headaches, depression and anxiety, which all fall under the umbrella of neurological conditions.

Just as confirmation of diabetic and metabolic support was uncovered in 2014, lavender's neuroprotective abilities were confirmed time and again in 2012 – the year of the lavender! In other words, science and history are slowly but surely meeting on common ground.

A full literature review made its way to the *International Journal of Psychiatry in Clinical Practice* in 2010, confirming lavender's efficacy over the breadth of seven separate trials. A lavender essential oil capsule under the name Silexan was shown to consistently relieve symptoms such as sleep disturbance, anxiety, and low quality of life. What's more, no one reported side effects, interactions, or withdrawal symptoms. If you've ever encountered pharmaceutical use for these conditions, you know how incredible that statement is!

Lavender's neuro-heroics don't stop with sleep. Research confirms time and again its incredible properties.

• A 2012 study conducted in Germany demonstrated the

restorative benefits of inhaled lavender essential oil vapor. With 60 minutes a day inhaled by rats with **dementia**, lavender was shown to prevent scopolamine-induced oxidative stress. (4)

- The same study took Post Traumatic Stress Disorder into consideration, as well, finding significantly improved sleep, moods and health, as well as reduced depression in individuals who were plagued with PTSD.

- In the same year, *Complementary Therapies in Clinical Practices* published a control study that highlighted the benefits of lavender for postpartum women. Twenty-eight women at high risk for postpartum depression found lessened **anxiety and depression** symptoms under a four week lavender aromatherapy treatment plan. (5)

- Finally, in 2012, *Molecules* took a different neurological route when they published the theory that lavender may be a treatment worth considering for **stroke**. Yes, you read that right! According to the study, *"In comparison with the model group, treatment with lavender oil significantly decreased neurological deficit scores, infarct size, the levels of [free radical], and attenuated neuronal damage [and antioxidants]."* (6)

Lavender as an Antimicrobial Agent

As much as lavender has been inhaled for neurological health, it has been utilized as an antimicrobial protectant against infections and disorders. Nearly one hundred studies have been conducted and published on this topic, confirming repeatedly what history has known to be true.

Generational wisdom has rarely used oils singly when treating infectious illness. The combination of oils creates a synergistic reaction, maximizing each oil's potential. This has been validated with science.

Scientists from the University of the Witwatersrand, South Africa found that 75.6% of the forty-five blends they attempted produced favorable results. Of the blends used, the *lavender-cinnamon* and *lavender-orange* mixtures were the most powerful. *Candida albicans* and *Staph aureus* were susceptible to a 1:1 ratio of these oils, both frequent causes of topical and respiratory illness. (7)

Lavender Soothes and Heals the Skin

Those antimicrobial and antioxidant components come full circle in this last – and certainly not least – major benefit of lavender essential oil.

Particularly when mixed with a soothing carrier oil like aloe or coconut – 10 drops per 1 ounce – lavender is highly effective against sunburns, dry skin, minor scrapes and cuts, and canker sores. Even some immediate-type allergic reactions may be mitigated with lavender! (8, 9)

As part of a calming, soothing salve for daily use, lavender blends well with sandalwood essential oil.

Lemon

And dulling tastes of happy Citron fruit,
Than which, no helpe more present can be had,
If any time stepmothers worse than brute
have poyson'd pots, and mingled herbs of sute
With hurtfull charmes: this Citron fruit doth chase
Blacke venome from the body in every place.

~ Virgil 70 BC – 19 BC

Despite the quote from the storied author above, the history of *Citrus limon* is quite silent. The lemon itself is native to Asia, grown from a small, evergreen tree. Multiple cultures claim the lemon as their own, from Burma and China to northeast India. Botanists from the University of California have their own twist, believing that the lemon is actually a hybrid fruit, combining sour orange and citron, rather than standing alone as a historical species. (1)

So while we speak so frequently about the historical use of many essential oils, the history of lemon itself is shrouded in mystery and uncertainty. We have seen lemons in Ayurvedic medicine for as much as a century, and lemons appear again in Josephus' writings, describing a high priest's *fruitful* encounter with an angry crowd in 90 B.C. – who preceded to pelt him with lemons for his errant ways!

Lemons in Ayurvedic Tradition

Traditional use has carried us where historical origins fail, and we have plenty of record of lemon's benefits in Ayurvedic medicine, followed in recent decades by scientific confirmation.

Ayurvedic food and medicinal preparations use lemon and lemon essential oil heavily, giving us an excellent basis for discovery and use.

Assistant professor of Alva's Ayurveda Medical College, Dr. J.V. Hebbar, relays the **13 key benefits of lemon in the Ayurvedic model:** (2)

1. Vakrashodhi – Oral health
2. Rochana – Digestion.
3. Trushna Nivarana – Thirst quencher.
4. Shula Nivarana – Remedy for abdominal colic pain.
5. Kasa Nivarana – Cough relief.
6. Kaphotklesha, Chardi Nivarana – Calms stomach and relieves nausea, excessive salivation and vomiting.
7. Amadoshahara – Prevents malabsorption.
8. Hrutpeeda – Relieves chest pain due to gastritis.
9. Asya vairasya hara – Relieves bad breath
10. Vahnimandyahara – Promotes digestion, it is a naturally detoxifying.
11. Varnya – Improves complexion and skin tone.
12. Pushtiprada – Nourishes the skin.
13. Kapha Dosha – Weight loss.

Other notable effects include the regulation of cholesterol deposits in the circulatory system, which can help to reduce risk factors for heart disease!

Current Research on Lemon Essential Oil

Hundreds of studies have referred to lemon essential oil, exploring the dozens of traditional uses. Its most prominent component, limonene, is likely the key to its potency, found in many citrus oils but none so strongly as lemon. Its cancer-fighting antioxidant power is impressive, as well. With such a strong foundational composition, it's not surprising that the science is catching up to 1,000-year-tradition at breakneck speed!

One such study was released last spring (2014), highlighting the benefits that lemon essential oil has for pregnant women dealing with nausea and vomiting. One-hundred women participated, and after two days, stark differences were already noticed between the control group and those using lemon essential oil. Two days after that, lemon essential oil helped to decrease nausea by an average of 33%! (3)

Another component of lemon that researchers have recently validated is geraniol. To evaluate the antioxidant ability to reverse damage from inflammation and oxidative stress, scientists in India gave geraniol to rats with diabetic neuropathy. Over the course of the 8-week study, markers of sciatic nerve damage and mitochondrial enzymes were both restored significantly. As a bonus, they also observed restored dopamine levels, the neurotransmitter that is associated with healthy functions like movement and unhealthy functions like addiction. (4)

Although this was an animal study and not necessarily indicative of mirrored results in humans, the potential beneficial effects of regular lemon essential oil use are promising, especially with our current influx of mitochondrial disease and the effects of stress on the heart and aging. And, as concluded,

"From our data, we hypothesize that [geraniol] may be a promising therapeutic candidate in the management of [diabetic neuropathy] in humans!"

Food safety is another major benefit of lemon essential oil use. A USDA study utilized lemon in a study regarding *E. coli* and *Salmonella*. It successfully protected apple juice against the dangerous bacterial strains, confirming its antimicrobial use. (5)

After just a couple of examples, it already seems like lemon is a super-oil. And for good reason – it really is! Not only for us, but for our four-legged friends, as well. In 2014, Italian scientists documented the benefits of bitter orange, lavender, oregano, marjoram, peppermint, and helichrysum in a sweet almond/ coconut oil carrier on dogs with dermatitis. A common denominator and major active compound? Limonene. Twice daily applications for one month were comparable to conventional treatments, with no side effects and benefits lasting for six months. (6) Impressive, to say the least!

I would love to see the study replicated with lemon included or replacing some of the oils, since lemon contains the highest limonene amounts of all citrus oils. (7)

Fun and Effective Lemon Essential Oil Uses

We've already walked through quite a range of uses for lemon essential oil, so there's no surprise at the long list of practical applications. These are just a sampling, and some of my favorite ways to use lemon outside of medicinal benefits.

1. **Freshen Clothes** – We've all forgotten to switch laundry to the dryer at least once. Just add a few drops of lemon EO in a rinse to prevent that awful odor.
2. **Remove Gum and Sap** – Playtime around trees can quickly become a mess. Remove pine gum or tree sap from clothes and carpet with an essential oil application.
3. **Wash Greasy Hands** – Soap just doesn't always cut it after doing mechanic work. But with a couple of drops of lemon essential oil added to your soap, the grime should wash right off!
4. **Disinfect (Without the Toxins!)** – Alcohol and bleach are harsh, especially when little hands and lungs are around. Instead, add 40 drops lemon oil to 8 oz pure distilled water and 8 oz witch hazel or white vinegar to clean the moldy shower and germy countertops.
5. **Safe Leather Treatment** – A dab of lemon oil on a cloth will restore leather furniture, shoes, and clothing to their original luxe.
6. **Polish Silver** – Try the same effect on tarnished silverware and jewelry to bring back the shine.
7. **Goo-Be-Gone** – Sticker books are a parent's nemesis when the stickers find their home on windows and furniture. Remove

stickers, gum, and other gooey remnants with the help of lemon essential oil!

My family goes through 2-3 15ml. bottles a month! We enjoy a drop in our water, a few drops diffused, we clean with it, we take with some raw honey to give us an immunity boost. We love lemon essential oil!

What's YOUR favorite way to use lemon?

Lemongrass

In gardening circles, lemongrass is a beautiful ornamental grass that helps repel mosquitoes. In fact, whole "grass gardens" of intentionally grown grass meant for aesthetics are popping up, and lemongrass is a favorite. Outside of trendy garden spaces, lemongrass is a culinary staple in Thai cuisine as an herb with the intense flavor of – you guessed it! – lemons.

Originating in the East, lemongrass and its oils have been part of local traditions and medicine for decades. With the resurgence of essential oils worldwide and increasing popularity in the US, lemongrass essential oil has become one of the more popular choices in aromatherapy, and science is beginning to verify traditional uses and uncover its mechanisms of benefit – and lemongrass has a wide range of uses, from muscle pain to cosmetics.

Lemongrass Composition

Distilled from the dried blades of grass, Cymbopogon citrates has many chemical components that contribute to its beneficial actions. They include alcohols, ketones, terpenes, aldehyde, and esters. Many of these categories of chemicals are known for their very strong effects on the body – which is good news.

We see that strength play out in its many beneficial actions. To list a few, lemongrass essential oil has been studied for the following actions (1):

- Anti-inflammatory
- Antifungal
- Antimutagenic
- Antimalarial
- Antioxidant
- Antiparasitic
- Hypoglycemic
- Neurobehavioral
- Pain relief
- Lowering cholesterol

One of the first capabilities I look for is *antioxidant,* because that indicates an active healing effect. Antiodixants are often described as scavengers, searching for free radicals to stop and damage to reverse. Lemongrass stands among the antioxidant scavengers, making it an ally in all kinds of metabolic, chronic, and even cancerous illness. (2)

7 Healing Properties of Lemongrass Oil

Lemongrass essential oil is comprised of geraniol and neral, both found in other citrus-like essential oils. It exhibits a few properties pretty strongly, with a range of applications that extend from those benefits. Here are three actions that underscore lemongrass essential oil's strengths.

1. Anti-inflammatory

Inflammation can rear its ugly head in chronic illness, pain, skin conditions and more. It's one of the reasons researchers in Algeria took the time to evaluate lemongrass in 2014. They evaluated the results of a topical lemongrass essential oil preparation on mice for anti-inflammatory effects as well as antifungal effects (but we'll get to that in a minute). The results were clear enough that they noted lemongrass "clearly...inhibits the skin inflammatory response." (3)

2. Antifungal

In the same study, antifungal properties were examined as well, against multiple fungal enemies including the dreaded *Candida albicans*. With what may be a surprising twist, inhalation seemed to be the strongest application against candida. Final results were that lemongrass exhibits "noteworthy potential for the development of drugs for the treatment of fungal infections." In another study conducted a few years ago, in 2008, lemongrass showed "a potent in vitro activity against Candida." (4)

3. Antimicrobial

To take lemongrass from an antifungal for the body to a super-cleaning oil as well, lemongrass does in fact have antimicrobial benefits. For example, food scientists have been monitoring lemongrass for its ability to inhibit *Staph* and improve food preservation. In a study and a review, published in separate journals over the course of a year, lemongrass was viewed favorably as an option for food safety applications. (5, 6)

For you and I, this means lemongrass is a powerhouse in the cleaning department, especially in the kitchen and bathrooms where mold and microbes really take hold.

4. Combat Airborne Pathogens

Diffuse lemongrass with geranium to replicate 2009 efforts to mitigate airborne and surface bacteria in a UK study. They were able to reduce bacteria like MRSA and strains of resistant bacteria by as much as 89% through diffusion and sprays, declaring the oils to be successful disinfectants. (7)

Add lemongrass to DIY spray cleaners for kitchen counters to limit surface microbes and bacteria and for bathrooms to inhibit the growth of mold. Diffuse in the car and home for airborne disinfectant properties.

5. Anxiolytic

Folk use of lemongrass includes **antianxiety treatments**, and in 2011, scientists worked to confirm these effects. By evaluating neurotransmitters and their response to lemongrass exposure, they were able to track the way the body processes the oil. Their findings centered around the GABA receptors in the brain and confirmed an anti-anxiety reaction. (8)

Diffusion and inhalation are typically the best methods of administration for anxiety, providing an immediate access to the oil's properties. Add a drop to diffusers, air vents, or clothing for a steady stream of aroma, or make an inhaler of sorts by placing a drop on a handkerchief and breathing deeply when necessary.

6. Lowers Cholesterol

The journal *Food and Chemical Toxicology* published an article resurfaced a 30 year debate whether or not lemongrass oil can reduce elevated cholesterol levels with the following study:

"...one of the three experimental groups receiving lemongrass EO (1, 10 or 100mg/kg). No significant changes in gross pathology, body weight, absolute or relative organ weights, histology (brain,

heart, kidneys, liver, lungs, stomach, spleen and urinary bladder), urinalysis or clinical biochemistry were observed in EO-treated mice relative to the control groups.

Additionally,blood cholesterol was reduced after EO-treatment at the highest dose tested [~2 drops]. Similarly, data from the comet assay in peripheral blood cells showed no genotoxic effect from the EO. In conclusion, our findings verified the safety of lemongrass intake at the doses used in folk medicine and indicated the beneficial effect of reducing the blood cholesterol level." (9)

At roughly 2 drops per day, taking lemongrass essential oil is a superbly effective and simple approach to balance your cholesterol levels!

7. Cancer Killer

To date, 7 studies have evaluated lemongrass' potential connection with cancer. (10)

In 2009, a study was published that evaluated the essential oil from a lemon grass variety of Cymbopogon flexuosus for its in vitro cytotoxicity against twelve human cancer cell lines; as well as in vivo anticancer effects on mice. The results were quite promising, as researchers discovered various mechanisms of how the oil killed the cancer lines. "Our results indicate that the oil has a promising anticancer activity and causes loss in tumor cell viability by activating the apoptotic process as identified by electron microscopy." (11)

8. Bug Repellant

The lemongrass plant itself is often grown for **bug repellent** benefits, but the essential oil is much more portable! In trials just this year (2015), lemongrass matched DEET's performance for mosquito repellent, without all of those nasty chemical risks and side effects. (12) Add lemongrass to a water and vinegar mixture, shake, then spritz onto clothing for a DIY mosquito repellent.

As a side note, isn't it incredible that a plant native to the tropics of eastern Asia is also an effective antimalarial and mosquito repellent? The design inherent in nature and especially in the plant kingdom never ceases to amaze me – undoubtedly an indication of whose Kingdom we are really living in!

Safety Notes

As always, common sense and further education are always important when utilizing medicinal remedies and new topical treatments. Lemongrass is usually safe, but sensitive skin might react with discomfort and even a rash. Carrier oils can help to mitigate this, but always test (in a carrier oil) on a small area of skin first before going right to a massage. Also, internal consumption is safe and quite effective for most people if a therapeutic grade is used. To avoid esophageal irritation, take 1-2 drops in a gel capsule.

Myrrh

Gifted to the baby Jesus and remembered each year at Christmas, many of us may not realize that myrrh is actually used every day around the world. While most of our essential oils and herbal remedies come from leaves and flowers, myrrh is much more exotic. It is the resin, similar to a sap, of an African and Middle Eastern tree, the *Commiphora myrrha.*

We know that myrrh is of old thanks to the gifts of the Magi, but that's not the only documentation. **Ancient Egyptians**, as part of their intricate mummification process, utilized myrrh in their rituals. We have record from **Herodotus** that describes myrrh's use in approximately 450 B.C., though mummification was in practice for centuries prior. (1)

In other cultures, myrrh has been found historically used as medicine in **China** – still used to this day – as well as in Jewish anointing oils, no doubt among many other traditional uses for healing and ritual.

Myrrh essential oil is an incredible example of the way plant based medicines connect us with history. This tree has stood where ancient Egyptians and Hebrews walked, and still stands today, sharing its healing resin with yet another era. Not all healing is sweet and pleasant, though. Myrrh is named for the Arabic word for "bitter": murr.

Therapeutic Properties of Myrrh

Chemically, myrrh oil is comprised most notably of eugenol and terpenoids, both of which are known for their medicinal properties – for example, clove essential oil is comprised primarily of eugenol. (2)

Terpenoids have a reputation as potent healers, potentially because of their role in protecting the plant from oxidative stress. As we know, this kind of stress causes cell death, and it's not exclusive to humans. Terpenoids carry antioxidant capabilities, then, to ward of oxidative stress and preserve the plant. Fortunately for us, we can share that same preserving effect! (3)

After centuries of use in aromatic and medicinal forms, science is uncovering more and more of its benefits by the day. Some of the scientifically acknowledged properties of myrrh include:

- Antiseptic
- Anesthetic
- Antitumor
- Antiparasitic
- Antioxidant
- Wound healing

These actions have been traditionally applied to skin infections, oral health, inflammation, intestinal health, and pain relief, all confirmed in some way by modern science. (4)

The more research uncovers, the more we see stress in its various states as an underlying cause of so many illnesses and discomforts. It's no wonder that a powerful antioxidant would carry such varied benefits. And powerful it is! Myrrh exhibits an antioxidant effect strong enough that it can protect the liver – the "detox" organ that is bombarded with toxins every day – from oxidative damage. (5)

Not only does myrrh utilize antioxidant properties to seek out free radicals and reverse oxidative damage, but it may be able to eliminate cancer cells, as well. Researchers in China recently published their findings on myrrh's cancer fighting abilities, after lab tests demonstrated the inhibition of cancer cell growth. (6) As with most cancer research, the steps forward toward proven treatments are detailed and difficult, but the foundation is clearly there, and the potential is absolutely intriguing!

Myrrh in Healing Applications

So how exactly does one utilize such a powerful, ancient, even holy substance? Honestly, however you'd like! Myrrh has a well-studied background and has been demonstrated as one of the most effective remedies in more than one category. While it isn't so much an immunomodulator for illness prevention, its healing capabilities are quite possibly unmatched.

Antimicrobial Benefits — Microbes are all around us, in many shapes and forms both beneficial and deleterious. When we're thinking in terms of pharmaceuticals and traditional medicines, there are treatments for bacterial infections, another treatment for fungal infections, and still others for viruses. Prevention is compartmentalized, as well.

Natural antivirals, antifungals, and antibacterials exist, of course, with each substance carrying its own strengths and weaknesses. A strong antimicrobial, though, may have the ability to affect more than one category of microbes. Myrrh essential oil is one such antimicrobial substance. (7)

Wound Healing — With these antimicrobial effects in combination with pain and inflammation relief, myrrh is an excellent wound healer. In an interesting study evaluating postpartum women who delivered vaginally with an episiotomy, myrrh oil in a sitz bath or soap application was actually shown to help the perineum heal by warding off the identified bacteria Escherichia coli and Enterococcus faecalis. The researchers concluded, "These findings indicate that postpartum aromatherapy for perineal care could be effective in healing the perineum perineal care could be effective in healing the perineum." (8)

Oral Health — The mouth is a dirty place. We're exposed to so much through our mouths, making it a hotbed of microbes and potential illness. When we do get sick, our mouths often notice first – sore throats, phlegm, and other discomforts settle in as one of the first signs of many illnesses. What's more, diseases of the mouth and gums are all too common.

According to a review conducted by Egyptian researchers, myrrh "is one of the most effective herbal medicines in the world for sore throats, canker sores and gingivitis." (9) And when it is combined with frankincense essential oil, a special synergy occurs. According to a recent South African study,

"Frankincense and myrrh essential oils have been used in combination since 1500 BC...When assayed in various combinations, the frankincense and myrrh oils displayed synergistic, additive and noninteractive properties, with no antagonism noted. When investigating different ratio combinations against Bacillus cereus, the most favourable combination was between B. papyrifera and C. myrrha." (10)

Utilize its antiseptic, antimicrobial, and wound healing effects by putting a drop on your toothpaste when you brush your teeth each night.

Antiparasitic Actions — No one wants to think about parasite infestations, but what we really don't want is to be caught with a parasite and unable to treat it. Egyptian scientists tackled this issue, as well, working with patience who had signs of parasites in their stool. Antiparasitic treatments are often harsh and come with intestinal discomfort. After testing a treatment utilizing myrrh essential oil, "no signs of toxicity or adverse reactions" were a problem and the treatment was successful. (11) This was against a specific parasite, of course, but the potential for improved treatment and even protection against infection exists!

Cancer — Last, but certainly not least, the ability myrrh essential oil has in healing cancer is becoming a popular topic in the industry. One of the most thorough studies on the topic was published in the journal *Oncology Letters* in 2013, and this is what they discovered about frankincense and myrrh oils:

"The effects of the two essential oils, independently and as a mixture, on five tumor cell lines, MCF-7, HS-1, HepG2, HeLa and A549, were investigated using the MTT assay. The results indicated that the MCF-7 and HS-1 cell lines showed increased sensitivity to the myrrh and frankincense essential oils compared with the remaining cell lines. In addition, the anticancer effects of myrrh were markedly increased compared with those of frankincense, however, no significant synergistic effects were identified." (12)

Recommendation: For a truly Biblical combination, use frankincense and myrrh essential oils together for a synergistic blend of antimicrobial benefits!

Notably, these two resins are generally prescribed simultaneously in traditional Chinese medicine. They are used primarily to treat **blood stagnation** and **inflammatory diseases**, as well as for the relief of **swelling** and **pain,** (12) "A previous study identified that the combination of frankincense and myrrh oils exhibited synergistic effects on harmful bacterial infections *Cryptococcus neoformans* and *Pseudomonas aeruginosa*" (12, 13)

Oregano

How often have you heard – or even thought – *I'll just go in and get a round of antibiotics* – for an ailment of any sort? Usually, the physician concurs, and today's antibiotic of choice is prescribed. Childhood ear infections, cold symptoms, you name it.

The problem with automatic prescription of antibiotics, due to patient demand or physician ignorance, is that they are only effective against *bacterial* infections. If our illness is viral and we take an antibiotic, we're risking the loss of beneficial bacteria in our bodies and aiding the creation of bacteria-resistant superbugs, all with no healing benefit. Even when we are facing a bacterial illness, finding the right antibiotic is much more effective than prescribing a broad-spectrum antibiotic.

The Wall Street Journal brought this significant public health concern to light in a 2013 article about antibiotic overuse and misuse, stating: (1)

"Overuse of antibiotics, and prescribing broad-spectrum drugs when they aren't needed, can cause a range of problems. It can make the drugs less effective against the bacteria they are intended to treat by fostering the growth of antibiotic-resistant infections. And it can wipe out the body's good bacteria, which help digest food, produce vitamins and protect from infections, among other functions.

*In a July study published in the Journal of Antimicrobial Chemotherapy, researchers from the University of Utah and the CDC found that **60% of the time** physicians prescribe antibiotics, they choose broad-spectrum ones....*

A similar study of children, published in the journal Pediatrics in 2011, found that when antibiotics were prescribed they were broad-spectrum 50% of the time, mainly for respiratory conditions....

*Both studies also found that about **25% of the time** antibiotics were being prescribed for conditions in which they have no use, such as viral infections."*

Essentially, our current approach to prescribe broad spectrum antibiotics out of reflex is like sending the atomic bomb where the A-Team would have sufficed.

Natural Antibiotic Alternative

No, pizza is not going to cure your bacterial illness.

Medicinal grade oregano (*Origanum vulgare and Origanum majorana)* is grown in the Mediterannean, and its essential oil is extracted via distillation. Each pound of oil is a product of over 1,000 pounds of wild oregano, forming a potent and valuable medicine that has been valued for thousands of years and countless cultures.

Antibiotic Prowess

Most consumers have no idea that antibiotics come in multiple forms. Beyond the indication of broad-spectrum antibiotics, there are more qualifications that determine how an antibiotic is most effectively used – Gram-negative and Gram-positive bacteria are affected in their own ways, and certain antibiotics will be more effective against one than the other.

The *Journal of Medicinal Food* published an analysis of oregano oil's efficacy against three Gram-negative (*Escherichia coli, Salmonella typhimurium, Pseudomonas aeruginosa)* and two Gram-positive (*Staphylococus aureus* , *Bacillus subtilis)* bacteria. Medicinal, true oregano (*Origanum vulgare*) harvested at various growth stages were tested, and all three were effective against all five bacterial strains. (2)

Similar findings were published two years prior, when researchers in Pakistan found oregano oil to be effective against parasites and even cancer cells! (3)

With clear results against these common bacteria – especially the food safety-related *E. coli* and *Salmonella* – including oregano essential oil in meals seems wise for gastrointestinal protection and disease prevention.

Beyond Bacteria

We could go on for pages about the antibiotic effects of oregano oil, but there's more to it than that. Unlike pharmaceutical antibiotics that are essentially one trick ponies, oregano oil carries with it so many more benefits. It is truly the **ultimate natural treatment** and an answer to standard antibiotics.

Within the oregano essential oil extract, a phenol component called *carvacol* is arguably the reason that oil of oregano is so strong. When you search the PubMed database of peer-reviewed literature, carvacol is referenced in more than 800 separate returns. Researchers are intrigued by this component, to say the least.

Some of the conditions carvacol and oregano oil have been indicated for, aside from bacterial infections, include fungi, parasites, viruses, inflammation, cell death, tumors, pain, histamine reactions, and oxidative stress.

Carvacol stepped out among the crowd of medicinal components when the *European Review for Medical and Pharmacological Sciences* highlighted its ability to detoxify and protect against side effects caused by Methotrexate. (4)

For perspective, Methotrexate (MTX) is well known as dangerous but used anyway for its treatment capability in severe illness such as cancer and rheumatoid arthritis. The benefits outweigh the risks, but only just.

In order to measure the interaction between MTX and carvacol, MTX-treated mice were observed with and without carvacol. The anti-inflammatory effects were able to inhibit the negative effects of MTX.

Similarly, carvacol has also been shown to potentially, ""prevent pathogenic overgrowth and colonization in the large intestine during oral iron therapy" – a therapy for anemia associated with severe gastrointestinal complaints. (5)

The research that follows will be exciting to watch, because the implications of a natural remedy able to limit the effects of necessary prescriptions are vast. Beyond fascination, someone taking harsh treatments such as iron therapy or chemotherapy could face a very different future with the side effects controlled.

Practical Oregano Oil Use

After lambasting unnecessary use of antibiotics, then singing the praises of a powerful one, you are no doubt wondering what limits we should place on oregano oil and how it should be used properly.

At this point, we can't be sure, really.

Because of its potency and capabilities, oregano oil should be used carefully alongside the guidance of a natural health expert or naturally-minded health care provider. Always dilute it, and be sure to take orally in a gel capsule instead of straight with water.

If it's strong enough to tackle MTX, it's strong enough to be taken seriously. Seek out a natural health provider today and see how oregano oil might fit within your lifestyle and regimen.

Peppermint

No, we aren't talking about mints, gum, or candy canes. Really, it's quite fascinating – in a somewhat sad way – that peppermint is so commonly associated with sweet treats rather than medicinal benefits. Aside from lavender, peppermint may be the most versatile of all of our essential oil options. And yet we've limited it to Santa Claus and toothpaste.

Consider that peppermint has the ability to:

- Treat a variety of illness from stress and migraines to skin conditions to digestive wellness
- Combat cancer cells
- Remain gentle on the skin and body
- Affect the body via respiratory, digestive, or topical applications
- Remain affordable thanks to easy propagation
- Stand up to thorough research

Is there any reason at all that we wouldn't stock our cabinets with peppermint essential oil? Our culture is seriously missing out!

The History and Composition of Peppermint

Peppermint (*Mentha x peperita*) is a hybrid combination of watermint and spearmint that grows prolifically – in fact, it can take over like a weed. The aerial parts – flowers and leaves – are harvested for essential oil production, which is conducted via steam distillation. At this point, active ingredients typically include menthone at around 20% of the composition and menthol at roughly 40%. (1)

Typically, peppermint oil is used as an antiemetic (helps to prevent nausea) and antispasmodic (helps to prevent vomiting as well as any other harsh gastrointestinal contractions). It's a soothing digestive aid and beneficial during times of illness.

Historically, peppermint dates back as one of the oldest medicinal herbs used in Europe, an ancient remedy for both Chinese and Japanese cultures, and an Egyptian medicine in at least 1,000 B.C. When, in Greek mythology, Pluto pursued the nymph *Mentha,* he transformed her into an herb (guess which?) so that the generations to come would enjoy her just as well as he. Such a colorful legacy is contained well in this cool, accessible, effective substance.

Peppermint in the Literature

Stepping away from Greek literature and into the scientific realm, peppermint is found throughout databases of studies and reviews – even moreso when we look at its specific component *menthol.* With hundreds and literally thousands of mentions, scientists are all over this remarkable herb. I don't make promises and guarantees often, but peppermint is almost a sure thing: add it to your daily regimen and your life will never be the same.

Nausea Relief — For example, while we all hope to avoid surgery, sometimes it is a necessary part of life – and a common part of surgery is unpleasant post-operative nausea, to the tune of 1/3rd of surgical patients. In 2012, Clayton State University facilitated tests on peppermint essential oil's effects on this nasty phenomena. Moms who are in recovery from a Caesarean especially do not want to deal with vomiting and nausea on top of the mixed emotions of the joy of birth and pain of surgery, not to mention the time that could be spent bonding with their babies. So, moms were chosen for this study, with 35 respondents discovering "significantly lower" nausea levels with inhaled peppermint compared with standard treatments. ([2])

Irritable Bowel Syndrome — The use of essential oils is sometimes underestimated when limited to the connotations of "aromatherapy." Topical and occasionally internal applications are relevant, as well, and one drop mixed with one teaspoon of coconut oil or (internally) honey, rubbed on the stomach or ingested, can calm an upset stomach or indigestion in a snap. This remarkable ability is being broached by researchers, marked by a systematic review of the literature that cover's irritable bowel syndrome (IBS) and peppermint.

Nine studies were reviewed, spanning more than seven hundred patients, and the conclusion was clear – taking peppermint oil in enteric-coated capsules performs much better than placebo when it comes to pain and symptom management. In their conclusion, University of Western Ontario researchers stated that,

"Peppermint oil is a safe and effective short-term treatment for IBS. Future studies should assess the long-term efficacy and safety of peppermint oil and its efficacy relative to other IBS

treatments including antidepressants and antispasmodic drugs." (3)

Bug Repellant — One of my personal favorite benefit of peppermint essential oil is bug repellant — especially since I live in mosquito country!

In a comparison of seven commercial bug repellants, Terminix® ALLCLEAR® Sidekick Mosquito Repeller nearly topped the charts. If you aren't aware, this is an "all-natural" blend that lists cinnamon, eugenol, geranium, peppermint, and lemongrass oils. It was very close to a tie with OFF!®, the chemical-laden, DEET-filled commercial brand. (4)

Although I don't recommend Terminix® ALLCLEAR® because I have little faith in a big name company to use true, pure, therapeutic grade essential oils, the lesson is the same. It underscores the efficiency of essential oils, no matter their quality. And an effective essential oil blend most definitely is preferred to harmful, toxic chemicals or nasty 'skeeter bites!

Interesting Peppermint Essential Oil Uses

- **Ease Pain Naturally**– For a natural muscle relaxer or pain reliever, peppermint essential oil is one of the best. Try using it on an aching back, toothache, or tension headache.
- **Clear Sinuses** – Diffused or inhaled peppermint essential oil usually clears stubborn sinuses and soothes sore throats immediately. As an expectorant, the results may be long lasting and beneficial when you're down with a cold, plagued with a

cough, or struggle with bronchitis, asthma, or sinusitis.

- **Relieve Joint Pain** – Peppermint oil and lavender oil work well together as a cooling, soothing anti-inflammatory for painful joints.
- **Cut Cravings** – Slow an out of control appetite by diffusing peppermint before meal times, helping you feel full faster. Alternatively, apply a drop or two on your sinuses or chest to keep the benefits to yourself.
- **Energize Naturally** – Road trips, long nights studying, or any time you feel that low energy slump, peppermint oil is a refreshing, non-toxic pick-me-up to help you wake up and keep going without the toxins loaded into energy drinks.
- **Freshen Shampoo** –A couple of drops included in your shampoo and conditioner will tingle your scalp and wake your senses. As a bonus, peppermint's antiseptic properties can also help prevent or remove both lice and dandruff.
- **Ease Allergies** – By relaxing the nasal passages and acting as an expectorant, peppermint can help relieve symptoms during allergy season.
- **Relieve ADHD** – A spritz of peppermint on clothing or a touch on the nose can help to improve concentration and alertness when focus is needed.
- **Soothe an Itch** – Cooling peppermint and soothing lavender combine again to sooth an itch from bug bites or healing sun burns.
- **Block Ticks** – Stop ticks from burrowing with a touch of peppermint oil. Make sure you remove them by their head to lessen your chances of contracting Lyme disease!

Cautionary Common Sense

Be sure to follow professional recommendations, healthcare provider advice, and common sense when using peppermint essential oil. While it is incredible versatile and relatively gentle, it is still a medicinal-quality substance and should be treated with care. As with all oils, make sure to always dilute with a carrier oil and, as always, listen to your body and the wisdom of those who have used aromatherapy before us: essential oils are best in small doses!

Harvard Medical warns, peppermint essential oil can relax the esophageal sphincter and pose risks for those with reflux. Futhermore, they note a cautionary tale: *"Several years ago, Israeli doctors reported the case of a woman whose mouth and throat were chemically burned by the large amount of peppermint oil she took to treat a cold."* (5)

Taking one or two drops of peppermint in a **gel capsule** can remedy this risk relatively easily.

Rose

"An idealist is one who, on noticing that a rose smells better than a cabbage, concludes that it makes a better soup."

~ H.L. Mencken, A Book of Burlesques

Roses are so frequently associated with idealism. We wear rose colored glasses when we want to avoid the truth. A rosy disposition is unreasonably cheerful. The idioms don't originate with roses, of course – rose tinted glasses actually helped roosters not to fight! – yet there they are, circling back to this lovely flowering perennial family.

For those who practice natural medicine, roses are every bit as delightful and hopeful as they are depicted. Swedish chefs have added rose hips to soup as a centuries-old delicacy. Rose flower water has permeated culinary and folk medicine practice as long as we have had the ability to distill it – over a thousand years!

More than Just a Pretty Flower

The scent of roses evoke memories and emotions associated with young love and evening strolls through the garden. How many of us remember the first time we ate a rose? I do. It was awkward and I was uncertain – flowers are ornamental! Of course, you wouldn't walk through a random garden (and certainly not a nursery or flower shop!) to pick a rose for dinner, but the organic, edible petals were pleasantly delicious. Why had I never done this before?

Later, rose essential oil hit my radar and I was fully hooked. You see, more than their beautiful blossoms and sweet smell, roses are a live-giving source of nutrients and healing.

Healing Properties of Rose Essential Oil

Distilled from *Rosa* damascene petals, rose essential oil carries a myriad of chemical compounds that bring wellness and healing to the body. Just some of the properties include:

- *Citronellol* – Known for its contribution to citronella, its most popular feature is as an effective mosquito repellant.
- *Citral* – Part of vitamin A synthesis, citral is found in lemon myrtle and lemongrass as well, and is a strong antimicrobial agent.
- *Carvone* –Also found in dill and caraway, carvone acts as a digestive aid.
- *Citronellyl Acetate* –This is where roses get their pleasant aroma, and is a key component of beauty products and fragrances.
- *Eugenol* –Found most richly in clove, which is likely the most powerful antioxidant substance in existence.
- *Farnesol* – A safe and natural pesticide, farnesol is found in ylang ylang, jasmine, and orange blossoms as well as rose essential oil.
- *Methyl Eugenol* – A component of lemon balm and cinnamon, it has local antiseptic and anesthetic effects.
- *Nerol* – Hops and lemongrass also boast this antibiotic with a gentle, sweet aroma.

- *Phenyl Acetaldehyde* – Yet another sweet scent, this compound is shared with chocolate!
- *Phenyl Geraniol* – Geraniol is often found in flavorings and perfumes, but this is the natural form.

With so many well-studied compounds contained in these delicate petals, it is little wonder that rose is so beneficial! *Rosa damascena* reportedly contains the most of these chemicals compared with other rose varieties, as well as a stronger fragrance.

Health Concerns Addressed By Rose Oil

How wonderful is our God to place such rich and powerful healing effects in a beautiful and fragrant package! With the most attractive flowers and fragrances emerging as some of the most beneficial, just think of all the good that colorful, fragrant, and beautiful fruits, vegetables, and edible flowers can impart in your diet! The abundant life is a lovely one, and rose essential oil you experience it by addressing these 3 health concerns.

1. Depression – The first example that comes to mind when describing rose essential oil's effects would be its interaction with depression. Imagine struggling against a dampened mood, faltering mental state, or all out depression. Now place yourself in our ancient ancestors' shoes, with nature more readily accessible, and the wild sights and sounds of flowers surround you. Are you drawn to the flowers? Do you inhale the fragrance and take the moment in, a twinkle in your eye? Like magic, some of that heavy load begins to life.

Better than magic, it's science!

The draw to beautiful flowers and fragrances went under the figurative microscope as published by the journal *Complementary Therapies in Clinical Practice*. Clinical tests of nearly thirty women in a postpartum stage of life treated half of them with a rose and lavender oil aromatherapy treatment. They followed this practice twice weekly for a month, while the control group did not. Remarkably, postnatal depression was lessened in the rose group, as well as a lower occurrence of anxiety! (1)

Recommendation: Place a diffuser by your bed, and enjoy 5 drops each of lavender and rose essential oils before bed. Rest, and allow the therapeutic benefits to work as you sleep.

2. Antimicrobial - Skin Health — Really, multiple components of rose essential oil make it ideal for skin treatments. Chinese researchers in 2010 pinpointed an excellent reason to include a few drops in DIY lotions and creams. In their studies, they found rose essential oil to contain some of the most potent antibacterial effects out of ten essential oils evaluated. After five minutes at just 0.25% dilution, rose essential oil was able to completely destroy the bacteria that causes acne (*P. acnes*). (2)

More evidence of rose's benefits for the skin emerged from Germany, also in 2010, not for what it could eliminate but for what it could create. Researchers explained that, *"For substances applied in rose oil a clear relationship between their lipophilic character, chemical structure, and skin permeation could be confirmed." (3)*

In other words, rose helps to drive substances into your skin, increasing permeability and carrying with it whatever it contains. For natural preparations, this is an excellent trait. For toxin-laden commercial products that happen to include *Rosa damascene,* you may be ushering the worst right into your body!

Recommendation: Truly clear acne by dapping one drop of pure rose essential oil directly onto blemishes when they arise, continuing three times a day until it is gone. For safe application, use a sterile cotton swab, and dilute with a bit of coconut oil if preferred.

3. Relaxation & Heightened Libido – Bringing rose oil home may be more romantic than the roses themselves. As an effective anti-anxiety oil, stress and anxiety related sexual dysfunction may be relieved with rose essential oil. According to a study published in the journal *Neuropsychiatric Disease and Treatment* that evaluated the effectiveness of various treatments have on SSRI-induced sexual dysfunction (SSRI-I SD) for men with major depressive disorder (MDD),

"This double-blind, randomized, and placebo-controlled clinical trial showed that the administration of R. damascena oil ameliorates sexual dysfunction in male patients suffering from both MDD and SSRI-I SD. Further, the symptoms of depression reduced as sexual dysfunction improved!"

Recommendation: Planning a lovely evening with your spouse? Use the bedside diffuser for two drops each of rose, sandalwood, jasmine and ylang-ylang. OR, to take things up a notch, place the oils in almond or jojoba carrier oils and gift your partner with a massage. The massage will be heightened by the aromatic, relaxing, and sensual fragrances.

Rosemary

"As for Rosmarine, I lett it runne all over my garden walls, not onlie because my bees love it, but because it is the herb sacred to remembrance, and, therefore, to friendship; whence a sprig of it hath a dumb language that maketh it the chosen emblem of our funeral wakes and in our burial grounds."

~ Sir Thomas More (1478-1535)

We love rosemary on potatoes and chicken, but it's so much more than a culinary treat. *Rosmarinus officinalus* was a sacred substance for nearly all ancient peoples, including Egyptians, Hebrews, Greeks, and Romans. As an evergreen Mediterranean native, rosemary would have been readily available, so its presence in folk medicine over the centuries is unsurprising.

Ancient peoples used rosemary for many purposes, including:

- Mental clarity
- Digestive soothing
- Muscle pain relief

In recent uses, rosemary is frequently used in skincare and hair products thanks to known antiseptic ability. As with many ancient remedies, rosemary is the subject of modern research as we begin to unlock the medicinal wisdom of generations past.

Can Rosemary Treat Cancer?

Although we only have in vitro (cells in a petri dish) studies, researchers suggest that rosemary essential oil can help prevent and treat a variety of cancer cells lines. Of the 30 compounds in the essential oil, there are a few main players: α-pinene, borneol, (−) camphene, camphor, verbenone, and bornyl-acetate. Interestingly, it doesn't seem that any one of these chemicals is responsible for rosemary's anti-tumor prowess. The research actually suggests that it's the synergy of them interacting together, which gives rosemary essential oil the true medicinal effect.

The study suggesting this was published in the journal Molecules after evaluating in vitro antibacterial activities and toxicology properties. of R. officinalis L. essential oil compared to α-pinene, β-pinene, and 1,8-cineole. According to the study,

"R. officinalis L. essential oil possessed similar antibacterial activities to α-pinene, and a little bit better than β-pinene, while 1,8-cineole possessed the lowest antibacterial activities. R. officinalis L. essential oil exhibited the strongest cytotoxicity towards three human cancer cells. Its inhibition concentration 50% (IC50) values on SK-OV-3, HO-8910 and Bel-7402 were 0.025‰, 0.076‰ and 0.13‰ (v/v), respectively. The cytotoxicity of all the test samples on SK-OV-3 was significantly stronger than on HO-8910 and Bel-7402. In general, R. officinalis L. essential oil showed greater activity than its components in both antibacterial and anticancer test systems, and the activities were mostly related to their concentrations." (1)

Four Favorite Benefits of Rosemary

Alongside the exciting prospect of slowed cancer growth and inflammation spread, rosemary has effects that are useful for our more common needs as well. Here are four of the ways rosemary exhibits its strengths in our everyday lives.

1. Hair Growth

Stimulating for the scalp, rosemary is a dandruff and dry scalp treatment that may facilitate hair growth. Some even go as far as to say that it can prevent hair loss and graying.

Years ago, Francesc Casadó Galcerá patented a lotion for scalp and hair (*US 6447762 B1*), including a mixture of rosemary, hops, and swertia. H found that his blend was able to stimulate (2):

- New hair growth, by as much as 22%
- Stimulated "rapid" hair growth
- Improved scalp health via microcirculation
- Smoother hair
- Retained hair, with fewer incidences of loss after shampooing

Include rosemary essential oil in simple vinegar hair rinses or DIY shampoo and conditioner formulas for improved scalp health and hair growth.

2. Memory Retention

"There's rosemary, that's for remembrance, pray you love, remember.

~ Ophelia (Shakespeare's "Hamlet")

Rosemary has been known as the "herb of remembrance" for centuries. Greek scholars used it when taking exams to help recall important information, and allusions to its memory improvement have been peppered into poetry throughout the ages. The *International Journal of Neuroscience* published one study that confirmed these effects in recent science.

Over 140 participants were gathered for the study conducted by University of Northumbria, Newcastle. Aromatherapy including rosemary and lavender, as well as a control group were utilized to affect cognitive performance.

- Regarding lavender and it's calming abilities, *"lavender produced a significant decrement in performance of working memory, and impaired reaction times for both memory and attention based tasks."*
- On the other hand, as a memory stimulant, *"rosemary produced a significant enhancement of performance for overall quality of memory and secondary memory factors."*

In other words, lavender made participants feel relaxed and complacent, while rosemary increased alertness and provoked memory retention. (3)

Test taking and alert feelings pale in comparison to the studies conducted on rosemary in relation to Alzheimer's disease. One such study, published in *Psychogeriatrics*, evaluated the effects of aromatherapy on 28 elderly people suffering from dementia, with the majority also diagnosed with Alzheimer's disease. They were given rosemary and lemon inhalations in the morning, then lavender and orange in the evening. Through multiple tests and forms of analysis, the "patients showed significant improvement in personal orientation" without any deleterious side effects. (4)

3. Liver and Gallbladder Support

The primary function of the liver is to detoxify the body, and with such heavy levels of toxins exposed to us on a daily basis, sometimes it can use a little help.

Traditional use of rosemary includes digestive and gastrointestinal relief. (5) Coupled with liver support, rosemary becomes a fantastic detoxifier. This has been confirmed in studies conducted in India, where it was observed helping the body increase its bile production and improve plasma liver enzyme levels. When these processes are inhibited, fat metabolism and detoxification are inhibited, and risks for type II diabetes increase.

With a properly functioning liver, gallbladder, and gastrointestinal system, nutrients are more readily absorbed and toxins released, bringing balance and wellness to the whole body.

4. Reduced Cortisol Levels

The Meikai University School of Dentistry in Japan conducted a study that monitored cortisol levels in saliva after just five minutes of rosemary and lavender inhalation. Twenty-two volunteers participated, and both essential oils had excellent results. Not only was the "stress hormone" cortisol reduced significantly, but free radical scavenging activities were increased as well. (6) So the oils help to prevent added stress, then go a step further to help erase effects of previous stressful exertion.

Implementing Rosemary Uses

Clearly a safe and effective oil, rosemary's benefits can be implemented in many ways. Here are just some of my favorite DIY recipes for application:

- **Aromatherapy Use** – Add 5 drops to your favorite diffuser, which typically contains four ounces of fluid.
- **Dietary Supplementation** – Dilute 1 drop in a teaspoon of honey, maple syrup or coconut oil.
- **Culinary Use** - Next time your recipe calls for rosemary, add a drop or two and experience a Heavenly burst of flavor!
- **Topical Application** – Enjoy its antioxidant and antiseptic properties on the skin, but be sure to heavily dilute with coconut, almond, or jojoba oil before applying to skin.

Sandalwood

One of the most recognizable fragrances in aromatherapy, sandalwood is used most widely in the perfumery industry to the tune of hundreds of tons of oil each year. In Eastern cultures, sandalwood appears in holy ceremonies and religious rituals. It marks significant events like weddings and births, as decorations and ceremonial rites.

Derived from the *Santalum* genus, sandalwood trees have been grown all over the world. Usually, *Santalum album* out of the Indonesian region is the most commonly utilized species for essential oil production. Outside of that region, the US carries the highest demand for sandalwood, and it has been increasing, driving the price up, as well.

It's an evergreen tree grown for the heart wood, which is harvested after heavy rains once the tree is a certain size. The inner wood is powdered, then steam distilled for essential oil extraction. With increasing demand meeting a difficult cultivation process and potentially unsustainable harvesting practices, we could ultimately lose sandalwood altogether. (1)

Sandalwood Composition

The maturity of the tree at harvest and the depth of color affect the specific composition of the essential oil that is extracted. Of the molecules that comprise sandalwood, the most notable is *santanol,* making up 80-90% of the sandalwood essential oil. (2)

If harvested too young, the santanol amounts will be on the lower end, affecting the expected medicinal properties. When using sandalwood, it's important to trust your source, both to know what to expect from it and to trust them to use ethical and sustainable methods.

Health Properties of Sandalwood Oil

While many essential oils come from the leaves and flowers of plants and, therefore, share similar components, sandalwood is different. It comes from the heart of the tree and boasts primarily varieties of santalol molecules. Still, they are powerful substances, and the beneficial effects aren't decreased in the lack of variety.

1. Sedative Effects

Traditional Asian remedies often include sandalwood for anti-anxiety effects, and science is confirming these abilities. In 2011, researchers from Japan isolated santalol to observe its effects on the CNS system of rats. After administration, they monitored sleep, motor activity, and other components of relaxation, ultimately confirming santalol and sandalwood's traditional sedative use. (3)

2. Antioxidant Ability

As with many essential oils, sandalwood carries strong antioxidant abilities. One major benefit of antioxidant substances is their effect on metabolic conditions, as noted by a 2013 study published in the journal *Phytomedicine* that evaluated the antioxidant benefits of diabetic mice. They concluded that, *"it was observed that the beneficial effects of a-santalol were well complimented, differentially by other constituents present in sandalwood oil, thus indicating synergism in biological activity of this traditionally used bioresource."* (4) What other constituents sandalwood contains, santalol brings out the best in them!

3. Alternative Anti-Inflammatory

Also related to metabolic and chronic illness, inflammatory conditions are pervasive in our country. Last summer, Canadian scientists took pure *a*-santalol and *b*-santalol extracts and weighed them against ibuprofen's abilities. The results were so promising that they called for topical applications as a comparable anti-inflammatory agent. (5)

4. Skin Tonic Abilities

Sandalwood oil carries several properties that are beneficial in skin care, from antiviral properties protecting against infectious intruders, to antiseptic abilities to help keep skin clean and clear. (6, 7) Its significant astringent ability helps to tighten and freshen skin, as well.

5. Anticancer Potential

In lab tests, sandalwood essential oil seems to exhibit protective abilities against various kinds of cancer cells. (8) The journal

Carcinogenesis detailed the potential that sandalwood and santalol show when, in 2004, a study demonstrating skin cancer cell growth inhibition and death (apoptosis) thanks to *a*-santalol. (9) Prostate cancer cells met a similar fate in 2012's *Phytomedicine* edition, again showing apoptosis by *a*-santalol. (10) Whatever researchers uncover about essential oils and potential cancer prevention and treatment, I'm certain that I want these substances in my body if cancer cells were ever to try to crop up!

Some Other Ways to Use Sandalwood

Because of the overuse and underproduction of sandalwood, we must use extra caution to not only source it well, but to use it well. Such clear health benefits cannot be ignored, so integrate sandalwood into your wellness routine with care and respect for our natural resources. Here are some go-to ways to use sandalwood and maximize its effect.

Reduce Anxiety

We've already seen its sedative effects, and small sample tests have shown promising anti-anxiety results from massage. (11) Just a small amount of sandalwood essential oil can help to calm anxious, restless nerves in any situation. Not only do I recommend it for relaxation when it's time to sleep, but anxious situations may benefit from its calming effects, as well. For a quick, DIY diffuser, add a drop or two to the air conditioner vents of your car to circulate the stress relieving ability.

Clean House

As an antiseptic and antiviral, utilizing sandalwood in cleaning and home diffusion may help to minimize the disease-causing substances in your home. The herpes simplex virus, even drug resistant strains, is susceptible to sandalwood – along with thyme, which is another excellent antiviral oil (12) – as is the flu virus! Beta-santalol (*b*-santalol) comes to the forefront in this case, when Indian researchers demonstrated significant success against influenza strains, prompting further research into essential oils and the flu. (13) Include a few drops of sandalwood in your DIY cleaning preparations to inhibit viruses, or diffuse throughout the home to clear the air, particularly when you have lots of interaction with others who may bring viral exposure.

Treat and Protect Skin

Make the most of antiseptic, astringent, and protectant effects of sandalwood by including a drop or two in your lotion and cleanser preparations. As a potential skin cancer protective agent, especially consider it on facial remedies, since our faces are exposed to so much sun on a daily basis.

While sandalwood has been reported in rare cases of reaction or sensitization, overall it is proving itself as a safe oil with antimicrobial and anticancer benefits setting it apart. (14) Use common sense and caution as with any other oil, but pay extra attention to sourcing and frivolous use that may threaten this wellness gem.

Tea Tree

One word spoken by the World Health Organization (WHO) has rocked the health world, confirming what natural health practitioners have warned us about for years: *superbugs*.

The overuse of antibiotics and antimicrobial treatments is creating drug resistance, a public health threat in which bacteria, a fungus, or a virus can become completely resistant to drugs – a superbug that can withstand all treatment. The WHO statement on superbugs cautioned,

This means that standard treatments no longer work; infections are harder or impossible to control; the risk of the spread of infection to others is increased; illness and hospital stays are prolonged, with added economic and social costs; and the risk of death is greater—in some cases, twice that of patients who have infections caused by non-resistant bacteria. (1)

As terrifying as this prospect is, it is becoming more reality than science fiction, and we have very little time to act to prevent it.

A Public Health Crisis

When traditional medicines are taken for their antibiotic, antiviral, and antifungal effects, far more than the targeted concern is destroyed. The gastrointestinal system probably fares the worst, with beneficial microbial life disrupted. To restore balance, energy and healing efforts are directed toward this damage, taking away from other healing and wellness efforts. Essentially, a spiral of insufficient gut flora reduces immunity, diverts restorative energy, and weakens the body, which is then susceptible to more infections that would need more treatment, and the cycle goes on. You can see how superbugs can quickly become lethal.

Superbug *H041* is a sexually transmitted disease that was discovered by public health officials in Japan in 2011. Researchers and natural health professionals agree that this is a frighteningly dangerous health threat. Professor Cathy Ison of the National Reference Laboratory for Gonorrhea expects that it will become untreatable soon. (2) Health officials in the US called for over $50 million in immediate education and awareness funding to help mitigate the dangers of *H041*. (3)

This is just an example of superbug transmission that should concern us even if we aren't practicing unsafe sex, because it demonstrates the capability superbugs have to threaten public health.

What are health care officials left to do?

Should they allocate more money to engineer even stronger, more potent antibiotics that will inevitably become useless or – worse- enhance the problem as bacteria evolve permanent resistance? Or, in a novel approach, could Congress approve measures to fund research toward the best ways to use natural, established, effective solutions like essential oils? I see much more long term potential in

102| Using God's Medicine for the Abundant Life!

the latter, and here are some of the reasons why.

Tea Tree Oil as a Natural Antibiotic

Melaleuca Alternifolia hails from Australia, used as a traditional remedy on the eastern coast for centuries. Crushed tea tree leaves soothed cuts and wounds in medicinal poultices. Inhaled vapors treated respiratory illness and discomfort. Finally, in 1923, tea tree oil's antiseptic benefits were scientifically validated when Arthur Penfold discovered the essential oil was a dozen times stronger than carbolic acid!

With this knowledge in hand, Australians brought tea tree oil with them as they fought in World War II. Around this time, pharmaceutical antibiotics came on the scene, disparaging the use of natural remedies. Just a few short years after Western science proved the efficacy of a centuries old traditional remedy, the same science threw it by the wayside. In the '60s, the disdain was so heavily felt that the tea tree oil industry collapsed completely, only recently making its return to global popularity.

Results of Current Research

Slowly, science is catching up in explaining why tea tree oil is such an effective antimicrobial agent. Over three hundred studies are returned referring to tea tree oil's antimicrobial benefits. We know that centuries of use were warranted, but now we are seeing reasoning for *Melaleuca's* effectiveness in traditional remedies for conditions such as:

- Acne
- Bacterial infections
- Chickenpox
- Cold sores
- Congestion and respiratory tract infections
- Earaches
- Fungal infections
- Halitosis
- Head lice
- Psoriasis
- Dry cuticles
- Insect bites, sores and sunburns
- Boils from staph infections

And this list doesn't even include the cosmetic and general home uses of tea tree oil, such as make-up removal, laundry freshening and deodorizing.

Returning to its basic foundation as an antibiotic, a 2013 *Phytomedicine* study weighed the safety factors involved with taking essential oils alongside traditional antibiotics. The essential oils, including tea tree oil, were safe and free of adverse reactions taken in conjunction with popular antibiotics ampicillin, piperacillin, cefazolin, cefuroxime, carbenicillin, ceftazidime and meropenem. What's more, the synergistic effects that we love so much with combined essential oils sometimes occurred with the antibiotics, potentially helping to prevent some resistance. (4) If you absolutely must take an antibiotic course, it may be beneficial to add tea tree oil alongside it.

If it were up to me and some researchers, the antibiotics would never be up for use in the first place. Tea tree oil demonstrated itself as fully effective against *Staphylococcus aureus*, *Streptococcus sobrinus*, *Streptococcus mutans,* and *Escherichia coli* in a recent study out of Taiwan, with additional benefits as an anti-inflammatory agent. (5)

Not only does this indicate a promising natural alternative to antibiotics in terms of resistance, but as an affordable remedy, it is a cost effective solution, as well.

Caution and Reassurance

As with any strong oil, potency should be considered with regard to safety, and some have suggested that tea tree may be toxic and too strong to use. Officially, thanks to a study out of the *Journal of Ethnopharmocology*, researchers have deemed it safe to use, just as centuries of wisdom and use have indicated. (6) Simple antibiotic safety principles should be observed, such as confirming bacterial infection before treatment, using only what you need, and taking in gel capsules.

Thyme

A perennial that can bunch up as a bush or creep along a forest floor, thyme is a ground cover, soil nutrient, and "living mulch." Really, thyme is similar medicinally to its botanical presence: it's always there, sturdy and without much fanfare, but accomplishes important things.

To obtain the essential oil, the leaf and flower of *Thymus vulgaris*, or garden thyme, are steam distilled. Named either for its strong, herbaceous fragrance (*thymon* – to fumigate) or its association with bravery (*thumon* - courage) , thyme's "roots" reach back to ancient Greece.

Analyzed for its chemical properties, thyme essential oil is comprised of a component called thymol, followed by gamma-terpinine and cymene. Thymol is most studied, with a rash of research covering its food safety and antimicrobial benefits. (1) In fact, it stands out as thyme's most notable function, cleansing of microbes and danger. Once again, thyme's presence in the botanical world mirrors that of the essential oil realm. As a plant, it grows along the surface of the ground, preventing moisture loss and protecting the soil and the plants around it. As an essential oil, thyme continues it protective mission, cleansing surfaces and the air around it of detrimental microbes and fungal invasions.

The plant world is teeming with these complete packages of nourishment and health! When we fill our homes and lives with naturally protective substances like thyme, along with its fellow nourishing, healing, and relaxing foods, herbs, and essential oils, we add benefits to our whole life – mind, body, and spirit!

Mechanism of Benefit

You've made it this far into the book, but I'd be willing to bet that the chemical names and composite structure of an essential oil is probably still not what you're looking for. Unsurprisingly, the technical details rarely hold interest – we want to get right down to the meat of things. What can we DO with the components? For thyme oil, some of the possibilities are pretty promising!

Immunostimulant — While thyme protects us as an antimicrobial for cleaning and food safety, which we'll look closely at in a moment, it may also help condition us to respond to microbes we encounter. The *International Immunopharmacology* journal published a study in 2014 that demonstrated thymol, a main substance in thyme essential oil, as a white blood cell stimulant and immune-boosting substance. (2) We all talk about health from the inside out, but thyme may be single handedly embodying that philosophy!

Antidepressant — One avenue that thymol appears to take in the body is through neurotransmitters associated with depression. Published in *Behavioral Brain Research* this year (2015), Chinese researchers followed the effects of thymol on "chronic unpredictable mild stress," observing anti-inflammatory relief on the neurotransmitters that cause depression. Its potential as an antidepressant therapy is exciting and one I'm looking forward to seeing discovered and developed. (3)

Anticancer — In a previous chapter, we looked at a study that demonstrated the benefits rose oil carried against acne bacteria. In the same study, cancer cells were also evaluated to see how they could stand up against ten powerful essential oils. Thyme was one of those oils, and it stood out from the crowd as most beneficial against the cells of prostate, lung carcinoma, and breast cancers. (4) While it can't be stated enough that these studies are preliminary, I'm filled with hope for a future where naturally occurring products replace toxic chemicals for cancer treatment and – dare we hope? – cures!

Balancing — As one of the top herbs for estrogen binding, thyme may be able to help the body balance and regulate hormones. (5) Incidentally, this is not the only time we have seen a potential estrogenic herb noted for its anticancer potential, as well. Because cancer frequently holds receptors for estrogen, thus being fed by anything estrogenic, we often suggest avoiding estrogen if you have or are at high risk for cancer. But with potent anticancer potential, we may one day find that what we thought were cancer-causing plants and foods were really giving our bodies a blueprint for fighting cancer on its own!

Some Practical Uses

Anti-fungal — In a study released this year, thyme joined lemon, basil, geranium, clove, and cinnamon as highly effective against fungi, including *Candida albicans* and the resulting candidiasis. (6) Antifungal properties are important as a cleaning agent, but I'm especially interested in tools to battle systemic Candida struggles. This specific study occurred in vitro (in lab tests), but we have seen other studies demonstrate inhalation as an effective essential oil application against Candida. Diffuse a couple drops each of thyme, cinnamon and clove for a spicy, herbaceous fragrance that can help ward off Candida.

Antibacterial — Thyme is an excellent addition to cleaning solutions, with potent antimicrobial properties. To establish antibacterial control in potentially one of the most infections environments – a commercial chicken house – Polish scientists used essential oil mists and monitored the antibacterial results. Both peppermint and thyme mixed with water were tested separately for three days, with both exhibiting strengths against specific bacteria. (7) Combining antimicrobial and antibacterial oils helps to facilitate that incredible synergistic effect that feels like magic – with each oil enhancing the abilities of the other. Diffuse thyme, peppermint, and lemon for an energizing and disinfecting effect. Add to a spritz bottle for topical disinfecting, particularly in the kitchen after handling raw meats and other food safety risks.

Food Safety — Thyme is especially well utilized when we take advantage of its antimicrobial prowess and improve food safety. Commercial applications are intriguing, with the potential for preservation and packaging to occur with natural substances like thyme oil. But safety in our homes is important, as well.

For example, a chicken marinade using thyme and orange essential oils was able to inhibit *Salmonella*. (8) A 2004 study and 2007 study found similarly beneficial effects against *Listeria* and *E. coli,* respectively. (9, 10) Though we should all be practicing good kitchen hygiene and food safety habits anyway, including thyme oil in food preparations may help to make up for shortcomings commercially – if nothing else, it's a bit of added peace of mind!

Citrus Oils

Citrus fruits are like the sunshine of the produce world. They are colorful and bright, fresh and juicy – the perfect sign that summer is here. Their essential oils bring a similar cheer, whether cooking, cleaning, bathing or simply breathing, citrus oils can be part of the process, refreshing and revitalizing along the way.

While most essential oils are produced via steam distillation, citrus oils are different. The leaves, bark, roots, and seeds aren't the source of the oil – it's the fruit itself! More specifically, the peel of citrus fruit provides the essential oil. If you've ever been sprayed in the eye when peeling an orange, or felt the oily residue on your fingers afterward, you've encountered a citrus essential oil already.

To produce citrus essential oils, the peel is usually cold pressed, extracting the oil without the application of heat or solution, otherwise called "expression." The peels can be steam distilled or extracted with a solution, though they are less common methods, and the latter is known as an absolute rather than an essential oil and is not used in the same ways. (1)

A note to remember about citrus oils: we often think of foods with thick peels as less dangerous when grown conventionally because the peel protects the edible part from toxic pesticides. The opposite is true in this case. The peel is in constant contact with sprays, so the concentrated essential oil product would be, as well.

Always trust your essential oil provider to bring you toxin and residue free oils!

Shared Composition of Citrus Essential Oils

Since we are looking at an entire family of fruits and their essential oils, shared features are to be expected. The most prominent and noteworthy component of citrus oils is *limonene*, confirmed in a study evaluating multiple citrus oils for their ability to improve food safety via antimicrobial effects. (2)

Another commonly shared chemical is *bergapten*, notable for its phototoxic effects. When bergapten is left on the skin, then exposed to the sun, it amplifies the effect of the sun and can leave burns. Some people like to avoid using bergapten-heavy oils topically altogether, but simply avoiding the sun after use (such as using it at night before bed) is sufficient. Alternatively, steam-distilled citrus oils have lower concentrations of bergapten and mitigate this effect. The citrus oils that contain bergapten when cold pressed are bergamot, lemon, and lime. The others are safe for normal use. (3)

With shared **antimicrobial benefits**, citrus oils are almost universally good in cleaning formulations. But each has its own strengths, and there is room in the oils cabinet for all of them!

Citrus Oils for Everyday

There are few things citrus oils cannot remedy. From the countertop to your intestines, they clean, detoxify and are wonderful additions to any home!

Bergamot

Officially named *Citrus Bergamia,* bergamot differs from the other citrus oils in that it's not a familiar fruit. In fact, it's not even an edible fruit in any practical sense. Still, its oil has been used for some time now, flavoring black tea and appearing in traditional Chinese remedies.

Bergamot essential oil is an important oil for **stress relief**. In one very recently published study coming out of Japan, mood, cortisol levels, and fatigue were all relieved in a short amount of time after inhaling bergamot essential oil. (4)

Another strong benefit of bergamot is its **antibacterial activity**, not only good for surface cleaning but also implicated in **food safety**. Researchers are focusing heavily on citrus oils to inhibit *E. coli* and other bacteria, and bergamot is one of the most promising. (5)

Grapefruit

The grapefruit is an undersold tool for **weight management**. If you struggle with maintaining a healthy weight, no doubt you've seen grapefruit recommended in every diet, from the healthier "eat well" varieties to the dangerous crash diets. That's because every part of the grapefruit is good for your metabolism and body composition, right down to the essential oil.

One mechanism of the benefits may be connected to an internal reaction to the scent, that basically tells the body it's time to burn fat. (6) Topically, massages including grapefruit oil have shown reduced cellulite and body circumference, as well as increased self esteem. (7) There are internal benefits, as well, though it should be noted that doses are quite important – no essential oil should be taken in high quantities, regardless of recommendations from friends, family, or blogs. Always consult with a professional, especially when weight management is the concern and goal.

Lemon

We've already looked in-depth at lemon essential oil and its benefits for the body. Lemon contains the highest levels of limonene, the active component that brings us most of the benefits from citrus oils. Aside from the benefits for ourselves, limonene and lemon essential oil are excellent options for DIY cleaning recipes. Limonene is so beneficial, in fact, that commercial cleaning products synthesize it for their formulations! (8)

Use lemon essential oil in sprays for countertops, faucets, doorknobs, and any other surface that comes into contact with germs for a **strong antimicrobial, protective effect**.

Lime

Lime essential oil is quite similar to lemon in composition, which makes it an effective option for cleaning as well as for synergistic blends. A noteworthy finding on its cleaning abilities, lime essential oil was shown to be an effective surface antifungal in addition to its **antimicrobial** effects. (9)

For the body, combine lime with other citrus oils in diffuser blends to boost their combined benefits. Cleanse the air, energize your spirits, and lift your mood with the bright scents and powerful composition.

Orange

Orange essential oil can be found as sweet, bitter, or wild, depending on the variety of the plant and the time of harvest. The components and fragrance will vary between each, but at least one component is shared among them – orange oil is the most commonly studied and used oil for food safety. One in particular blended orange with thyme to marinate chicken, finding significant protection against *Salmonella* growth. (10)

Recommendation: *Add one drop of a citrus oil to a tsp of honey, maple syrup, and/or coconut oil then mix with morning water or afternoon tea for a refreshing pick-me-up, spritz down counters with citrus oil and vodka blends where food preparation occurs, and marinate dinner with a citrus oil infusion. In other words, citrus oils should be used daily!*

Conclusion

The thief comes to steal, kill and destroy. I have come that they may have life and have it abundantly!

~ John 10:10

I hope you have enjoyed this journey down the road of evidenced-based essential oil uses. If you haven't tried them yourself, I strongly encourage you to give them a try. As God's Medicine, you won't be disappointed if you give your medicine cabinet a makeover!

Essential oils are a wonderful way to take charge of your own health, and determine in your heart to learn more about natural solutions and remedies to everyday problems. Please visit my website at www.DrEricZ.com and stay current with my essential oils database. Let's encourage one another to never settle and always strive to learn more about how to best honor our bodies as the temples of the Holy Spirit. And don't forget to leave a comment or two. We're all on this journey together!

Shalom!

~ **Dr Z**

References

Top 10 Essential Oils for Healing

1. http://www.essentialoils.co.za/history-essential-%2520ils.htm
2. http://www.ncbi.nlm.nih.gov/pubmed/24031950
3. http://www.ncbi.nlm.nih.gov/pubmed/24262758
4. http://www.spandidos-publications.com/ol/6/4/1140?wptouch_preview_theme=enabled
5. http://www.ncbi.nlm.nih.gov/pubmed/24373672
6. http://www.ncbi.nlm.nih.gov/pubmed/24066512
7. http://www.ncbi.nlm.nih.gov/pubmed/26072990
8. http://www.webmd.com/vitamins-supplements/ingredientmono-644-oregano.aspx?activeingredientid=644&activeingredientname=oregano
9. http://www.ncbi.nlm.nih.gov/pubmed/23537749
10. http://www.ncbi.nlm.nih.gov/pubmed/24269249
11. http://www.ncbi.nlm.nih.gov/pubmed/23513742
12. http://www.sciencedirect.com/science/article/pii/s0378874113008490

Clary Sage

1. http://www.bibliomania.com/2/1/66/113/frameset.html
2. http://pubget.com/articles/elasticsearch_show/0671f940-3eaa-4e28-80af-2502b3a89296
3. http://www.tandfonline.com/doi/abs/10.1080/10412905.1999.9701074#.VbEjG_lVg_8
4. http://pubget.com/articles/elasticsearch_show/24929006
5. http://www.ncbi.nlm.nih.gov/pubmed/24835194
6. http://www.ncbi.nlm.nih.gov/pubmed/10071073
7. http://pubget.com/articles/elasticsearch_show/25672419
8. http://www.ncbi.nlm.nih.gov/pubmed/25821423
9. http://pubget.com/articles/elasticsearch_show/23157022
10. http://www.ncbi.nlm.nih.gov/pubmed/20441789
11. http://www.ncbi.nlm.nih.gov/pubmed/21949670,
12. http://pubget.com/articles/elasticsearch_show/22435409
13. http://www.ncbi.nlm.nih.gov/pubmed/11033651
14. http://www.ncbi.nlm.nih.gov/pubmed/24802524

Clove

1. http://www.superfoodly.com/orac-values/
2. http://www.superfoodly.com/orac-value/spices-cloves-ground/
3. http://www.ncbi.nlm.nih.gov/pubmed/24099633
4. http://www.ncbi.nlm.nih.gov/pubmed/24031950
5. http://www.ncbi.nlm.nih.gov/pubmed/15720571

6.   http://www.ncbi.nlm.nih.gov/pubmed/16530911
7.   http://www.ncbi.nlm.nih.gov/pubmed/22997520

Eucalyptus

1.   http://www.ncbi.nlm.nih.gov/pubmed/24831245
2.   http://pubs.acs.org/doi/abs/10.1021/np400872m
3.   http://www.ncbi.nlm.nih.gov/pubmed/22860587

Frankincense

1.   http://www.hindujagruti.org/hinduism/knowledge/article/why-do-we-light-lamp-in-front-of-deities-in-the-evening.html#11
2.   http://www.ncbi.nlm.nih.gov/pmc/articles/PMC3538159/
3.   http://www.ncbi.nlm.nih.gov/pmc/articles/pmc1112084/
4.   http://www.ncbi.nlm.nih.gov/pubmed/22171782
5.   http://www.ncbi.nlm.nih.gov/pubmed/?term=frankincense+essential+oil+cancer
6.   https://www.mskcc.org/cancer-care/integrative-medicine/herbs/beta-elemene
7.   http://www.ncbi.nlm.nih.gov/pmc/articles/PMC3796379/
8.   http://www.ncbi.nlm.nih.gov/pubmed/18167047
9.   http://www.indianboswellia.com/pdf/prof_ammon_research.pdf
10.   http://www.ncbi.nlm.nih.gov/pubmed/25312172
11.   http://www.ncbi.nlm.nih.gov/pubmed/25312172
12.   http://www.researchgate.net/publication/270275886_frankincense_as_a_potentially_novel_therapeutic_agent_in_ovarian_cancer
13.   http://www.biomedcentral.com/1472-6882/9/6
14.   http://www.ncbi.nlm.nih.gov/pubmed/22171782
15.   http://www.ncbi.nlm.nih.gov/pubmed/23850473
16.   http://www.oapublishinglondon.com/article/656
17.   http://www.ncbi.nlm.nih.gov/pubmed/23500016
18.   http://www.ncbi.nlm.nih.gov/pubmed/22066019
19.   http://www.ncbi.nlm.nih.gov/pubmed/21287538

Helichrysum

1.   http://www.ncbi.nlm.nih.gov/pubmed/18606217
2.   http://www.ncbi.nlm.nih.gov/pubmed/24239849
3.   http://aac.asm.org/content/53/5/2209.long
4.   http://www.ncbi.nlm.nih.gov/pubmed/22799105
5.   http://www.ncbi.nlm.nih.gov/pubmed/23140115
6.   http://www.ncbi.nlm.nih.gov/pubmed/15507345
7.   http://ghqscul.ishib.org/ED/journal/20-1s1/ethn-20-01s1-78.pdf

Lavender

1.   http://www.ncbi.nlm.nih.gov/pubmed/22895026

2. http://www.sciencedirect.com/science/article/pii/s0944711312005120
3. http://www.ncbi.nlm.nih.gov/pubmed/24373672
4. http://www.ncbi.nlm.nih.gov/pubmed/22475718
5. http://www.ncbi.nlm.nih.gov/pubmed/22789792
6. http://www.ncbi.nlm.nih.gov/pubmed/22895026
7. http://www.ncbi.nlm.nih.gov/pubmed/23737850
8. http://www.ncbi.nlm.nih.gov/pubmed/22558691
9. http://www.ncbi.nlm.nih.gov/pubmed/10217323

Lemon

1. http://journal.ashspublications.org/content/126/3/309.full.pdf
2. http://easyayurveda.com/about/
3. http://www.ncbi.nlm.nih.gov/pubmed/24829772
4. http://onlinelibrary.wiley.com/doi/10.1002/jnr.23393/abstract
5. http://www.ncbi.nlm.nih.gov/pubmed/15366861
6. http://www.ncbi.nlm.nih.gov/pubmed/15366861
7. http://www.perkinelmer.com/cmsresources/images/app_lim

Lemongrass

1. http://www.ncbi.nlm.nih.gov/pmc/articles/pmc3217679/
2. http://www.ncbi.nlm.nih.gov/pubmed/15796587
3. http://www.ncbi.nlm.nih.gov/pubmed/25242268e%20uses!
4. http://www.ncbi.nlm.nih.gov/pubmed/18553017
5. http://www.ncbi.nlm.nih.gov/pubmed/26147358
6. http://www.ncbi.nlm.nih.gov/pubmed/25280938
7. http://www.ncbi.nlm.nih.gov/pubmed/19292822
8. http://www.ncbi.nlm.nih.gov/pubmed/21767622
9. http://www.ncbi.nlm.nih.gov/pubmed/21693164
10. http://www.ncbi.nlm.nih.gov/pubmed/?term=lemongrass+essential+oil +cancer
11. http://www.ncbi.nlm.nih.gov/pubmed/19121295
12. http://www.ncbi.nlm.nih.gov/pubmed/25438256

Myrrh

1. http://pubget.com/articles/elasticsearch_show/11677605
2. http://www.researchgate.net/publication/ 10813073_components_therapeutic_value_and_uses_of_myrrh
3. http://www.ncbi.nlm.nih.gov/pubmed/16492481
4. http://pubget.com/articles/elasticsearch_show/17978635
5. http://www.ncbi.nlm.nih.gov/pubmed/19818824/
6. http://www.ncbi.nlm.nih.gov/pmc/articles/PMC3796379/
7. http://www.ncbi.nlm.nih.gov/pubmed/20922991
8. http://www.ncbi.nlm.nih.gov/pubmed/15314339
9. http://www.researchgate.net/publication/ 10813073_components_therapeutic_value_and_uses_of_myrrh
10. http://www.ncbi.nlm.nih.gov/pubmed/22288378

11. http://www.ajtmh.org/content/65/2/96.short
12. http://www.ncbi.nlm.nih.gov/pmc/articles/PMC3796379/
13. http://pubget.com/articles/elasticsearch_show/22288378

Oregano

1. http://www.wsj.com/articles/
   sb10001424127887323423804579023113596120826
2. http://www.ncbi.nlm.nih.gov/pmc/articles/pmc3868303/
3. http://www.researchgate.net/publication/
   260776284_composition_antioxidant_and_chemotherapeutic_prope
   rties_of_the_essential_oils_from_two_origanum_species_growing_i
   n_pakistan
4. http://www.ncbi.nlm.nih.gov/pubmed/24302176
5. http://www.ncbi.nlm.nih.gov/pubmed/24379194

Peppermint

1. http://www.ncbi.nlm.nih.gov/pubmed/19768994
2. http://www.ncbi.nlm.nih.gov/pubmed/22034523
3. http://www.ncbi.nlm.nih.gov/pubmed/24100754
4. http://www.ncbi.nlm.nih.gov/pubmed/23092689
5. http://www.health.harvard.edu/staying-healthy/
   understanding_and_treating_an_irritable_bowel

Rose

1. http://www.ncbi.nlm.nih.gov/pubmed/22789792
2. http://www.mdpi.com/1420-3049/15/5/3200
3. http://www.ncbi.nlm.nih.gov/pubmed/20225652
4. http://www.ncbi.nlm.nih.gov/pmc/articles/PMC4358691/

Rosemary

1. http://www.mdpi.com/1420-3049/17/3/2704?trendmd-shared=0
2. http://www.google.com/patents/us6447762?dq=rosemary+ess%2520ential
   +oil+hair+follicles
3. http://www.ncbi.nlm.nih.gov/pubmed/12690999
4. http://www.ncbi.nlm.nih.gov/pubmed/20377818
5. http://www.ncbi.nlm.nih.gov/pubmed/10641130
6. http://www.ncbi.nlm.nih.gov/pubmed/17291597

Sandalwood

1. http://www.fao.org/docrep/v5350e/v5350e08.htm
2. http://www.fao.org/docrep/v5350e/v5350e08.htm
3. http://www.researchgate.net/publication/
   242152600_variation_in_heartwood_oil_composition_of_young_sa
   ndalwood_trees_in_the_south_pacific_(santalum_yasi_s._album_a
   nd_f1_hybrids_in_fiji_and_s._yasi_in_tonga_and_niue)

4. http://www.ncbi.nlm.nih.gov/pubmed/23369343
5. http://www.ncbi.nlm.nih.gov/pubmed/24318647
6. http://www.sciencedirect.com/science/article/pii/s0944711399800464
7. http://www.ncbi.nlm.nih.gov/pubmed/19473851
8. http://ar.iiarjournals.org/content/35/6/3137.abstract
9. http://carcin.oxfordjournals.org/content/26/2/369.short
10. http://www.sciencedirect.com/science/article/pii/s0944711312001250
11. http://www.ctcpjournal.com/article/s1744-3881(05)00124-6/abstract
12. http://aac.asm.org/content/51/5/1859.short
13. http://www.sciencedirect.com/science/article/pii/s0944711311005319
14. http://www.sciencedirect.com/science/article/pii/s0278691507004309

Tea Tree

1. http://www.who.int/mediacentre/factsheets/fs194/en/
2. http://www.bbc.com/news/health-22263030
3. http://www.dailymail.co.uk/news/article-2319818/Sex-superbug-feared-worse-AIDS-discovered-Hawaii.html
4. http://www.ncbi.nlm.nih.gov/pubmed/23537749
5. http://www.ncbi.nlm.nih.gov/pubmed/24582465

Thyme

1. http://www.ncbi.nlm.nih.gov/pmc/articles/pmc4391421/
2. http://www.sciencedirect.com/science/article/pii/s1567576913004761
3. http://www.sciencedirect.com/science/article/pii/s0166432815003071
4. http://www.ncbi.nlm.nih.gov/m/pubmed/20657472/
5. http://www.ncbi.nlm.nih.gov/pubmed/9492350
6. http://pubget.com/articles/elasticsearch_show/25805904
7. http://ps.oxfordjournals.org/content/92/11/2834.full
8. http://pubget.com/articles/elasticsearch_show/24795320
9. http://www.sciencedirect.com/science/article/pii/s0309174007003853
10. http://www.sciencedirect.com/science/article/pii/s0309174007003853

Citrus Oils

1. https://www.naha.org/explore-aromatherapy/about-aromatherapy/how-are-essential-oils-extracted/
2. http://www.sciencedirect.com/science/article/pii/s0956713510003944
3. https://www.naha.org/explore-aromatherapy/about-aromatherapy/how-are-essential-oils-extracted/
4. http://www.ncbi.nlm.nih.gov/pubmed/25824404
5. http://www.ncbi.nlm.nih.gov/pubmed/17105553
6. http://pubget.com/articles/elasticsearch_show/15862904
7. http://www.ncbi.nlm.nih.gov/pubmed/17615482
8. http://pubget.com/articles/elasticsearch_show/3b99059e-6674-45be-b1a5-5607283c749a

9. http://pubget.com/articles/elasticsearch_show/3e26e320-b85e-46e1-ab59-57ea54cf9dcc
10. http://pubget.com/articles/elasticsearch_show/24795320

About the Author

Founder of DrEricZ.com, **Dr. Eric Zielinski** is a sought-after Biblical Health educator, author and motivational speaker. Inspired by the timeless principles in the Bible, Dr. Z's mission is to provide people with simple, evidenced-based tools that they need to experience the Abundant Life. By creating programs like Beat Cancer God's Way and hosting online events such as the Essential Oils Revolution and the Heal Your Gut Summit, Dr. Z educates people in natural remedies and empowering life strategies. He lives in Atlanta with his wife and three children.

Dr. Z Around the Web:

https://www.facebook.com/drericz
http://www.pinterest.com/drericz/
https://twitter.com/DrEricZielinski
https://instagram.com/drericz/

Made in the USA
Middletown, DE
30 March 2018